A History of Apprenticesh Training in Ireland

T0221357

In Ireland, as in many other countries, the education and training of nurses has undergone enormous change and has moved from what was a working apprenticeship towards a college-based professional education. *A History of Apprenticeship Nurse Training in Ireland* traces the progress of nurse education and training, presenting a new authoritative and scholarly account of the history of the traditional system of apprenticeship nurse training in Ireland.

Introduced as part of the reforms of hospital nursing in the late nineteenth century, apprenticeship nurse training was a vocational extension of secondary education and a form of paid employment for young women. It resided outside the mainstream of higher educational provision and provided nurses with the knowledge and technical skills for sick nursing. It also functioned to socialise them into the role of hospital worker and to inculcate in them nursing's value systems. This system of training provided a ready supply of skilled, efficient, inexpensive and loyal workers. With their 'bright faces and neat dresses', apprentice nurses were mostly young middle-class rural provincial women whose training experiences had features and functions of gendered education and gendered labour. Gerard M. Fealy exposes social, cultural, political and economic factors that have influenced the provision and reform of nurse training, and demonstrates how these factors have shaped modern nursing in Ireland. He also critically examines current historiography, bringing the hidden role of nurses and nursing to the fore.

Based on extensive primary sources, this in-depth study is essential reading for scholars and students of nursing history, women's history, and Irish social history.

Gerard M. Fealy is a nurse historian and a senior lecturer in nursing at the School of Nursing, Midwifery and Health Systems, University College Dublin. His research interests include the history of nursing and curriculum policy. Dr Fealy is the editor of *Care to Remember: Nursing and Midwifery in Ireland* (2005) and the co-editor of *Nursing Education in Drogheda, 1946–2004: A Commemorative History* (2004).

Routledge Studies in Nursing History

A History of Apprenticeship Nurse Training in Ireland
Gerald M. Fealy

A History of Apprenticeship Nurse Training in Ireland

Gerard M. Fealy

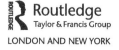
Routledge
Taylor & Francis Group

LONDON AND NEW YORK

First published 2006 by Routledge
2 Park Square, Milton Park, Abingdon, Oxon OX14 4RN

Simultaneously published in the USA and Canada
by Routledge
711 Third Avenue, New York, NY 10017

Routledge is an imprint of the Taylor & Francis Group

First issued in paperback 2012

© 2006 Gerard M. Fealy

Typeset in Baskerville MT by
GreenGate Publishing Services, Tonbridge, Kent

British Library Cataloguing in Publication Data
A catalogue record for this book is available from the British Library

Library of Congress Cataloging in Publication Data
A catalog record for this book has been requested

ISBN13: 978-0-415-35997-9 (hbk)
ISBN13: 978-0-415-65504-0 (pbk)

For
Deirdre, Mervyn and Jonathan

Contents

List of illustrations

Foreword

Read this narrative and realize once again how ubiquitous and essential modern nursing actually is. For more than one hundred and fifty years the idea and practice of nursing has spread across the world, transcending political boundaries and changing the experience of sickness and dependence. The idea of nursing was so formidable that it now seems that its expansion was inevitable. But, of course, no human endeavour is inevitable. Gerard Fealy offers us an invaluable and nuanced account of the reform called nursing as it appeared and developed in Ireland. As he does, he reveals nursing in its fullest context and creates the conditions for creatively and critically examining what *did* happen and what *is* happening in nursing and healthcare in our world today.

Viewing nursing through the lens of the state, religion, the economy and welfare schemes, we can see the intersection of motive and public priorities as the nursing reform developed in Ireland. We can also see how beliefs about health, gender and science shaped the course of change. Most dramatically, we can see that rising expectations placed on nurses by the public accelerated educational investment in nursing as the twentieth century drew to a close. The history of nursing in Ireland reveals once again how perfectly nursing mirrors the society it serves.

For international readers this history holds another special interest. For economic and social reasons Irish nurses have, for generations, migrated to every corner of the world. The impact of this nursing diaspora on the spread of nursing during the late nineteenth century and throughout the twentieth century has not yet been fully measured or understood. But the prevalence of Irish surnames on lists of nurses' names in many countries underscores the importance of migration. Our current recognition of the historic meaning of migration of people and ideas makes the Irish experience all the more compelling and relevant.

Finally, this history is a vital contribution to a still small but growing contemporary historiography of nursing. It is a major achievement which will move international historical scholarship forward. Most important of all, this book succeeds in conveying both the uniqueness and universality of the nursing reform experience in Ireland.

Joan E. Lynaugh, RN, Ph.D, FAAN
Emeritus Professor and Emeritus Director, Barbara Bates Center for the Study
of the History of Nursing, University of Pennsylvania, Philadelphia, PA, USA

Preface

As subject matter in the nursing curriculum in Ireland, history was usually allocated a few hours in the 'introductory block' and the topic typically consisted of an exposition of the history of the students' affiliated training hospital and some mention of the Crimean War. Lecturers' accounts of the history of nursing might begin and end with 'Miss Nightingale said ...', leaving the student with no real account of the historical development of nursing in Ireland, or with no sense that nursing in Ireland had its own unique history. Treating nursing history in this way reflected the more general indifference to history as subject matter in nursing scholarship and the somewhat marginalized position in which history as method and research programme has been located.

There is a deficit of published scholarship on the history of nursing in Ireland, and in the extant histories of Irish healthcare and related social history, nurses have remained largely hidden. Since much of what is published on the topic is found in the genre of amateur medical historiography, nursing history has tended to get subsumed into medical history and, in the process, has generally not been well described or has lacked a critical perspective. The aim of this book is to present an authoritative account of the history of the system of hospital apprenticeship nurse training in Ireland, from its inception to its demise. The book spans the period between the late nineteenth century, when apprenticeship nurse training emerged as an integral part of the reform of nursing in Ireland, and the late twentieth century, when the system ended with the entry of nurse training into the academy.

The book represents the fruits of doctoral research, which I undertook at the Education Department, University College Dublin. Through the rigour of historical method, I uncovered new evidence concerning the history of nursing in Ireland, and I also examined existing primary sources from a new *critical* perspective. In writing the book, I have endeavoured to present an integrated and inquiring historical narrative, which moves coherently through a series of interrelated themes that represent significant historical developments and/or chronological periods in the history of nursing in Ireland. The narrative is based on analysis and interpretation of documentary primary sources and is informed by the western European and American traditions of sociological and academic analysis, and by the international critical scholarship in the field. In this way, the book represents part of the new historiography of nursing. In my interpretations of primary sources, I have sought to expose underlying social, cultural, political and economic factors that influenced the provision and reform of nurse training in Ireland, and I have sought to demonstrate in an integrated way how these factors interacted to shape the development of modern nursing in Ireland. I have also endeavoured to demonstrate that while nurse training in Ireland was part of an international social practice, it had uniquely Irish expressions that were related to developments and activities in Irish social life and in Irish healthcare.

When the system of hospital apprenticeship training in Ireland ended in the 1990s, many commentators within and outside of nursing bemoaned the demise of the nurse apprentice and the passing of an era in which there appeared to be many more certainties in the professional lives and everyday work of nurses. This book reappraises the era of the nurse apprentice in the light of the new historical evidence.

I hope that the book will contribute an Irish dimension to international scholarship concerning the history of nursing and the training of vocational groups in Ireland and, in so doing, will provide a basis for international comparisons in social history in the areas of healthcare and professional-vocational education and training.

Gerard M. Fealy

School of Nursing, Midwifery and Health Studies, University College Dublin

April 2005

Acknowledgements

I am indebted to Dr Deirdre Raftery, my PhD research supervisor, for her guidance in the methods of historical research, her insightful observations and suggestions in the preparation of the historical narrative which forms the basis of this book, her genuine interest in and engagement with the subject, and her generous support and encouragement. I am also indebted to Professor Sheelagh Drudy for her leadership and encouragement.

I am indebted to the Examiners of the National University of Ireland for awarding me the Dr Mary L. Thornton Scholarship in Education, 2001. This scholarship provided me with affirmation of the worth of my research and it contributed in a significant material way to the research endeavour at the time.

I acknowledge the many individuals who provided me with encouragement and support during the preparation of this book. I extend my gratitude to Dr Marie Carney, Professor Pearl Treacy, and to all my colleagues at the School of Nursing and Midwifery, University College Dublin, for their encouragement, support and interest in my research. I acknowledge the support of the many librarians and archivists who provided advice and guidance to me in my pursuit of documentary materials during the course of my research. In this regard, I include mention of Mary Riordan and Peter Hickey and the other librarians at University College Dublin, Mary O'Doherty, Archivist at the Mercer Library, Royal College of Surgeons in Ireland, and Robert Mills, Librarian and Archivist at the Royal College of Physicians of Ireland. I also acknowledge the support of the librarians at Trinity College Dublin, the National University of Ireland, Maynooth, the National Library of Ireland, An Bord Altranais (Irish Nursing Board), the Irish Nurses' Organisation, and the Gilbert Library, Dublin. I am grateful to the many individuals who provided me with information on and access to primary source materials. These include Professor Seamus Cowman, Faculty of Nursing and Midwifery, Royal College of Surgeons in Ireland; Patrice O'Sullivan, former Principal Nurse Tutor, Mater Misericordiae University Hospital; Geraldine McSweeney, former Principal Nurse Tutor, St. Vincent's University Hospital; Josephine Leydon, former Principal Nurse Tutor, James Connolly Memorial Hospital; Barbara Garrigan, Director of the Centre for Nurse Education, St James's Hospital; and Anne-Marie Ryan, Chief Education Officer, An Bord Altranais.

I acknowledge the many international scholars who expressed encouragement and support. These include Susan McGann, Royal College of Nursing; John Adams, Homerton College, Cambridge; Claire Chatterton, University of Salford; Dr Margaret Currie, University of Luton; Dr Christine Hallett, University of Manchester; Dr Stephanie Kirby, University of the West of England; Professor Anne-Marie Rafferty, King's College London; Professor Peter Nolan, Staffordshire University; Malcolm Newby, Lincolnshire, and Dr Margaret Ó hÓgartaigh, Dublin. Other international scholars whom I wish to thank include Professor Mary Ellen Doona, Boston College; Professor Sioban Nelson, University of Melbourne; Professor Margaret Preston, Sioux Falls; Carol Helmstadter, University of Toronto; and the nurse historians at the University of Pennsylvania, most especially Professor Joan Lynaugh, Professor Pat D'Antonio and Professor Julie Fairman. I am also grateful to the American Association for the History of Nursing for embracing and supporting nurse historians in Ireland and, through their annual conference, for providing me with a forum to share some of the fruits of my research.

I reserve my deepest gratitude for my wife Deirdre and my children Mervyn and Jonathan for their unfailing love and support.

Introduction

While modern nursing in Ireland has origins in the religious-pastoral model of sick nursing proffered by Catholic sisterhoods in the early nineteenth century, the modern secular-professional nurse emerged as a result of an Anglican social reform movement in the late nineteenth century. Conducted initially in the Protestant voluntary hospitals in Dublin, nursing reform was led by members of the Anglo-Irish Protestant aristocracy, Anglican clergymen, Protestant medical men, and by a cadre of new Protestant nursing leaders who had received their nurse training in the reformed voluntary hospitals in England. In common with the reform of nursing in England, an integral part of the reform process in Ireland was the introduction of nurse training schemes based on the Nightingale model of hospital apprenticeship training.

In Ireland, hospital apprenticeship training prevailed for over 100 years as an intrinsic part of the country's health services. Since its inception, nurse training was more of the nature of paid employment for young women and less a form of higher education. As a vocational extension of secondary education, it resided outside the mainstream of higher educational provision. Hospital apprenticeship training aimed to provide the trainee with the knowledge and technical skills for sick nursing. It also functioned to socialize the apprentice into her role as a hospital employee and into nursing's value systems. It provided a ready supply of skilled, efficient, inexpensive and loyal workers. Entry to hospital training was the principal mode of entry to the nursing profession in Ireland, and the system of training rendered hospital nursing as the dominant model of sick nursing.

Aside from changes in the content of theoretical and clinical instruction, nurse training in Ireland remained largely unchanged for over 100 years. It also remained outside the mainstream of higher education long after the time when professional training for other healthcare disciplines had been assimilated into the academy.

This book presents a historical account of the system of hospital apprenticeship nurse training in Ireland, from the time of its introduction in the late nineteenth century to its demise at the end of the twentieth century. The book analyses and describes the development, provision and gradual reform of general nurse training, taking account of the social, cultural, political and economic factors that led to its initial establishment, its continuance, and its eventual disestablishment. In a chronological period spanning 115 years, the book explores a range of social developments that were directly and indirectly related to the development of nurse training in Ireland. Along this historical trajectory, the book narrates aspects of the policy and practice of nursing reform and aspects of the curricular experiences of the apprentice nurse, and it examines the principles and the values that gave rise to these experiences. The professional lives and the ideas of some of Ireland's most influential nursing leaders, including Margaret Huxley, are also examined. The narrative takes account of developments in scientific medicine and social policy in the nineteenth century, the women's movement, the emergence of the new Irish State and its efforts to provide a public health service, and international trends in healthcare and education. It also takes account of the fundamental changes that occurred in Irish public life with the transition from British rule to Irish independence.

Provision and reform

The social and economic changes occurring in the first half of the nineteenth century led to new relationships between rich and poor and resulted in the development of social policy that was aimed at the relief of poverty and the provision of medical relief. Chapter 1 describes these changes and examines the work of the principal providers of sick nursing in the period, the religious sisters, pauper nurses and untrained hospital nurses. These precursors of the modern nurse were of their time, but new developments in scientific medicine in Ireland had rendered them incapable of meeting the needs of either the medical man or the sick patient. This was especially true of untrained hospital nurses in the wards and clinical departments of the voluntary hospitals.

The bodies that provided and controlled the funding for the voluntary hospitals had enormous influence in hospital management policy, including nursing policy. Chapter 2 critically examines the role of two influential bodies, the Dublin Hospital Sunday Fund and the Dublin Hospitals Commission, in setting out clear policy on hospital nursing in the 1870s and 1880s. The chapter reveals the content of influential reports published by these bodies, which examined nursing arrangements involving untrained hospital nurses, and it describes the nursing policy that was developed at that time. The chapter explains the reasons why the two bodies in question were so influential in instigating a major process of nursing and sanitary reform in the late nineteenth century.

Using the historical case study approach, Chapter 3 examines the particular ways in which individual hospitals went about the process of nursing and sanitary reform, a process that included the introduction of new arrangements for the training of nurses. The chapter narrates the experiences of two Dublin hospitals as they underwent the transition from the old to the new system of hospital nursing.

By the early 1890s, nurse training in Ireland had attained its special characteristics in the Irish voluntary hospitals, such that recognizable common features were evident across the principal hospitals. Chapter 4 describes the curricular experiences of the early cohorts of young women who entered the new nurse training schemes in the Dublin hospitals in the 1890s, including their recruitment and selection, their conditions of employment, and their pedagogical experience. The chapter sets these experiences within the broader context of women's education in the late Victorian period.

By the early twentieth century, nursing leaders were actively campaigning for further reform of nursing, with the aim of attaining professional regulation through state registration. Chapter 5 examines the campaign for state registration in Ireland, identifying the conflicts and tensions in the campaign and the role of Irish nursing leaders in international developments in nursing in the period. The chapter also examines the role of the General Nursing Council for Ireland in the development of nurse training, highlighting its deliberations and policy decisions, and the ways that these decisions affected the nursing curriculum.

Chapter 6 examines the expressions of the curriculum in the general nurse training school in the years before and after state registration. The chapter comments critically on the principles of curriculum and instruction that gave rise to the range and type of curricular experiences provided in the period up to 1949, and it describes aspects of the organization and content of instruction. Some expressions of the hidden curriculum are also considered.

In 1950, as part of its strategy to develop a national public health service, the Irish Government established a new single regulatory authority for nursing and midwifery, An Bord Altranais (the Nursing Board). Chapter 7 explains the policy underlying the decision to establish the Nursing Board, and describes the changes brought about by the new Board in the areas of instruction and examinations. The chapter also discusses the curricular experience of student nurses during the years 1950 to 1979, examining classroom and ward learning experiences, as well as social aspects of the training experience.

Nursing policy in Ireland after 1980 was focused on the role of the nurse and on nurses' preparatory and continuing education and training needs. Chapter 8 evaluates the impact of this policy on the nursing curriculum, most especially the impact of European directives on the training of nurses. The chapter also analyses the political and professional debate that took place as a prelude to the dismantling of the system of apprenticeship training, and it considers the reasons why the system was discontinued in 1994.

The final chapter reprises some of the main conclusions in the book, and it analyses the process of change and reform as it pertained to nurse training in Ireland.

1 Charity, medical relief and precursors of the modern nurse

In the nineteenth century, the relief of poverty and the provision of medical relief were important expressions of Christian charity and the liberal ideals that emerged in the late eighteenth century. The relief of poverty and the provision of medical relief were organized and conducted by voluntary charitable bodies and increasingly by the state. The structures and activities associated with the provision of charity and state social services were the locus for interactions between rich and poor and represented the contexts within which the precursors of the modern nurse operated.

New social relationships

Begun in England at the end of the eighteenth century and occurring in Europe and North America in the nineteenth century, the Industrial Revolution brought new methods of commerce and advances in scientific knowledge and its application in engineering, manufacturing and medicine.[1] Industrialization brought changes in the methods of production, distribution and exchange, with the factory replacing the home as the principal source of manufactured goods. Industrialization was in turn accompanied by urbanization and the demise of the feudal system of social order and by great social and economic changes that affected most people's lives.[2]

In the new cities, new social structures emerged that were based on people's level of wealth and control of production and trade. In the move from a rural to an urban society, a new urban working class provided the labour that sustained the industrial development and wealth creation of the capitalist-employer or middle class, which comprised industrialists and merchants, and a cadre of new professionals, such as doctors, lawyers and bankers. While the Industrial Revolution brought enormous prosperity – so called 'new money' – paradoxically, industrialization and urbanization also brought much poverty. With the growth of cities, the urban labouring class experienced poor sanitation, poor health, and premature death from frequent outbreaks of infectious diseases. In Dublin and in many other Irish towns and cities, these problems were compounded by the arrival of displaced rural labourers fleeing the economic depression of the 1820s and 1830s and the Great Famine of 1845–1849.[3]

In the nineteenth century, the social interplay between the wealthy middle class and the urban poor was related to the economic division and the cultural distinction between the classes. The rich and poor led very different lives and differed in their thoughts and ideas, in their customs and religious practices, and in their public behaviour; in the view of Fredrich Engels, the working class were a 'race apart' from the bourgeoisie.[4] Aside from the workplace, the other principal areas of public life in which the rich and poor had contact was through the provision of public health and welfare services and through the giving and receiving of charity. The middle class was represented on political and administrative bodies, such as Parliament and the Poor Law Commission, and through these bodies, assumed responsibility for the well-being of the poor, intervening in their lives through legislation and a range of social welfare measures.

The social relationship between rich and poor was based upon the authority of the former and the subservience of the latter. It was given expression and strengthened in the enactment of legislation related to the relief of poverty and destitution, the provision of medical relief, and public sanitation. It was also expressed in humanitarian and philanthropic pursuits and in Christian charitable work.

Along with new relationships between rich and poor, new social relationships also emerged between men and women and between adults and children.[5] The intra-class relationship between middle-class men and women was given expression through ascribed roles in different spheres of life. Economic development led to a revision of the sexual division of labour; in theory and in practice, there was a recognized distinction between public life, the man's domain, and private life, the woman's domain.[6] This distinction was not stressed in the pre-industrial period, when women combined productive work, such as spinning and dressmaking, with domestic activity and childcare, and the 'woman worker' only became visible with the Industrial Revolution.[7] This visibility was constructed as a problem by nineteenth-century social commentators who pointed to the working woman's dilemma in having to combine domestic duty with paid employment.[8] The gender division of labour was offered as the rational, most efficient and most productive way to organize work, business and social life, and it set in opposition home and work, reproduction and production.[9] This division was a middle-class construction that not only separated domestic and public life, work and responsibilities, but also presented the woman worker as an anomaly, working in a sphere in which she did not naturally belong; this construction of roles according to gender was represented as the domestic and public spheres.[10]

Within each separate sphere came certain role expectations. In the domestic sphere, the middle-class woman's role was to be a wife and mother and to symbolize the wealth of her husband.[11] In the public sphere the man conducted business, commerce and politics. The middle-class woman was described as a 'gentlewoman' or 'lady', by which was meant she was not required to undertake menial work or to earn her living.[12] Freed from commercial productive responsibilities, her sphere of authority was concerned with maintaining domestic order, with the moral guidance and education of her children, and with the supervision of domestic servants.[13]

The middle-class woman derived her 'lady-like' status by acting out her ascribed role and, aside from writing and governessing, she could not work outside the home without the opprobrium of her class.[14] The pursuit of paid employment could lead to the loss of her status as a lady, and any foray into the public sphere could only take place for the purpose of charitable works.[15] These expectations brought with them considerable self-sacrifice, dependence on others and a high level of responsibility for the well-being of the family.[16]

For many women who aspired to a more fulfilling life, the home-centred existence could bring frustration and disenchantment. In her suburban home, the gentlewoman was constrained to live an idle domestic existence that included the supervision of servants and 'spending the day'. This latter activity was described in 1878 by Emily Davies, the campaigner for women's entry to higher education, as 'going to your neighbour's house at one o'clock and staying till ten, with nothing to do for the whole of those nine hours but sit and chat, with perhaps a bit of fancy work in your hand'.[17] Another activity which Davies described was that of 'receiving visitors'; this activity involved entertaining guests for several days or weeks, but it offered women little real stimulus or self-fulfilment:

> The process is wearisome enough for the guests, and terribly demoralizing to the poor hostesses, who conceive themselves obliged to hospitality to make this sacrifice of the order and continuity of their daily lives. By way of indemnity they return the visits, thus securing to themselves a double loss.[18]

Some outlets from this existence included essay and reading societies, but these activities offered little fulfilment. Many women needed more meaningful forms of self-expression and they needed an acceptable pretext for escaping the domestic sphere. Philanthropic pursuits and Christian charitable work offered such a pretext.

Philanthropy and Christian pastoral mission

In the nineteenth century, efforts at improving public health in Dublin included the appointment of the first Medical Officer of Health in 1864, the passing of the Sanitary Act of 1866, and the construction of a number of city sewerage schemes.[19] Despite these efforts, there was no significant decline in Dublin's death rate across the second half of the century and, for all its resident classes, the city was not a healthy place in which to live. The city's recorded death rate for the decade 1891–1900, at 29.65 deaths per 1000, was almost equal to that obtaining in the decade 1841–1850, when 30.13 deaths per 1000 were recorded.[20] Reasons why public health policy had little impact on the city's death rates included lax pursuit of sanitary policy on the part of public officials, financial constraints, and the political influence of vested interests, such as tenement landlords and slaughterhouse owners.[21]

The confluence of affluence and abject poverty in a city like Dublin and the prevailing humanitarian liberal ideals engendered a sense of social responsibility on the part of the wealthier classes.[22] This sense of responsibility was given practical expression through philanthropic work that included the establishment of charitable organizations. Middle- and upper-class Protestant women were especially active in charitable works aimed at alleviating suffering among the poor.[23] Philanthropic work in Ireland took a number of forms, including the building of institutions for the homeless and voluntary work in public institutions, such as workhouses, hospitals and prisons.[24] Philanthropy became especially important as an expression of social responsibility among the Anglo-Irish Protestant ascendancy.

Aside from its particular social function, philanthropy represented an acceptable alternative to paid work for middle-class gentlewomen, giving them a way of self-expression and a legitimate means by which they could enter the public sphere.[25] It permitted them to engage in extra-domestic pursuits without losing either their social status or the ladylike attributes of their ascribed role in promoting moral propriety and order; through charitable work, the middle-class gentlewoman could pursue her natural mission to ensure the spiritual and moral well-being of the poorer classes.[26] Visiting the homes of the poor to teach proper sanitation and participating on ladies' committees of voluntary hospitals were two expressions of the woman's mission.

Aside from philanthropic pursuits, the other principal means by which middle-class women could engage in extra-domestic work free from domestic responsibilities and expectations was through membership of a religious community. Membership of a religious community was an important means of self-empowerment and independence for middle-class women, and when combined with nursing, was seen as a legitimate extension of the woman's natural traits.[27] Related to moral and social imperatives concerned with improving the conditions of the poor, Christian pastoral missions were derived from the same humanitarian impulse that drove philanthropy. While the Reformation had caused a schism in the Christian Church, Christian charitable deeds remained at the heart of organized care of the sick in Europe, albeit from different interpretations of Christian duty; the Roman Catholic Church espoused care on the basis of Christian vocation, while the Protestant Church viewed care and charity as a social responsibility.[28]

The example set by European religious sisterhoods in France and Germany in caring for the sick best demonstrated the collective organization of Christian charitable work.[29] Inspired by religious vocation, evangelical mission and female piety, the French Catholic Daughters of Charity provided the inspiration and the model of sick nursing for the Catholic sisterhoods founded in Ireland in the early nineteenth century.[30] With a forthright evangelical mission, many of the new Christian sisterhoods that emerged in the nineteenth century acted to combine both physical and spiritual care of the sick.[31]

In England, the denominational care of the sick was conducted largely within the Protestant-evangelical tradition. Inspired by the Lutheran deaconess movement in Germany, a number of Anglican orders, including nursing orders, were formed in the nineteenth century.[32] They included the Society of Protestant Sisters of Charity, founded in London in 1840 by the philanthropist Elizabeth Fry, and the London Bible and Domestic Female Mission, founded in 1857 by the Christian evangelist Ellen Raynard.[33] Founded at St John's House by the Bishop of London in 1848, the lay Anglican sisterhood of the Order of St John the Evangelist provided a hospital nursing service to some of the principal London voluntary hospitals, and it also provided a home nursing service.[34] The St John's House order is generally regarded as being the first to establish a training school for nurses.[35]

While Catholic sisterhoods represented the largest group participating in denominational care of the sick poor in Ireland in the nineteenth century, there are examples of Protestant women engaging in evangelical and charitable work. A number of Irish bible societies existed as branches of English societies, but there were also indigenous Irish societies. These included the Dublin Visiting Mission (1859), the Dublin Bible Women's Mission (1861), the Young Women's Christian Association (1855), and the Girls' Friendly Society (1877). The work of these societies involved organized charity work on a large scale, and it included visiting the homes of the sick poor and establishing homes and schools for the destitute poor.[36] While the women of Protestant sisterhoods worked closely with male clerics, they were generally more independent of clerical authority than their Catholic counterparts.[37]

Following the repeal of the Penal Code in 1829, well educated Irish Catholic middle-class women found an outlet for personal fulfilment and religious conviction by engaging in charitable work as members of religious sisterhoods, and most prominent among these were the Sisters of Mercy and the Irish Sisters of Charity.[38] These new sisterhoods were made up of women from the wealthier Catholic families in Dublin. As the nineteenth century progressed, women of the poorer classes were admitted to the religious congregations, but they formed a servant class within their communities.[39] Like their Protestant counterparts, Catholic sisterhoods drew their inspiration from European religious orders. Founded by Mary Aikenhead in 1816, the order of the Irish Sisters of Charity was modelled on the French Filles de Charité. The French Soeurs de Charité provided the inspiration for the Congregation of the Sisters of Mercy, founded by Catherine McAuley in 1831.

Unlike their earlier monastic counterparts, these women did not lead a cloistered existence, but worked in the public sphere, principally in the areas of education and in the care of the sick poor.[40] As early as 1816, the Irish Sisters of Charity had begun to visit the sick poor in their own homes in Dublin and in 1833 they founded St Vincent's Hospital for the care of the sick poor in Dublin. The Sisters of Mercy provided a nursing service in the temporary hospitals that were set up in Dublin to cope with the Asiatic cholera epidemic of 1832.[41] Later they founded the Mercy Hospital in Cork in 1857 and the Mater Misericordiae Hospital in Dublin in 1861.[42] Through their extensive practical experience of sick nursing, the Irish Sisters of Charity and the Sisters of Mercy established new standards of nursing care, hygiene and hospital management.[43]

By the time of the outbreak of the Crimean War in 1854, it is evident that Catholic religious congregations, in particular the Sisters of Mercy, had developed considerable nursing expertise. In response to the call for nurses issued by the British War Office, Florence Nightingale and thirty-eight women travelled to the Crimea. Eighteen of this group were members of Anglican and Roman Catholic sisterhoods and five, whom Nightingale considered to be 'most excellent', were members of the congregation of the Sisters of Mercy from Bermondsey in London.[44] A second contingent of the Sisters of Mercy, a group of fifteen women led by Mother Francis Bridgeman from Kinsale in County Cork, travelled to the Crimea in December 1854.[45] This group played a little heralded but important role as military nurses in the Crimea; contemporary reports, along with later analysis of the personal diaries of some of the Sisters, indicate that their nursing system was superior to that proffered by the lay nurses under Nightingale.[46]

The denominational care of the sick offered by Catholic sisterhoods in Ireland was a part of society's response to the crises of poverty, epidemics, famine and increasing urbanization, a response shaped by what Sioban Nelson terms 'the Christian ethos that framed notions of service, pastoral care and community duty'.[47] According to Nelson, this same ethos contributed to the development of modern secular nursing in the way that it fostered imitation amongst secular women, including Nightingale and her contemporaries, such that the secular-professional model of nursing was an extension of and not merely a transition from the religious-pastoral model.[48] It may be that this imitation was quite literal, since history records that while hearing details from Mother Bridgeman of the system of nursing provided by the Sisters of Mercy in the Crimea, Nightingale took written notes.[49]

Throughout the nineteenth century, the institutional Catholic Church in Ireland, principally through the work of women's religious congregations, entered into partnership with the state in providing a wide range of social services, including education and sick nursing.[50] While initially directed at the poorer classes, this involvement became subject to 'social drift', becoming more oriented towards providing social services for the lower middle class.[51] By the second half of the nineteenth century, through their involvement in these services, Catholic religious congregations had successfully colonized the secular domain and had established a base of power and authority in Ireland that was instrumental in reshaping the social behaviour of Irish society well into the twentieth century.[52] Such was the extent of their involvement in providing nursing services in Ireland that nursing became closely associated with religious commitment in the public mind.[53] While Catholic sisterhoods provided a model for sick nursing, it would be lay Anglican women who would be instrumental in introducing modern secular-professional nursing into Ireland.

State social services: poor laws and medical relief

In the eighteenth century, poverty in Ireland was widespread and it was reported that 'strolling beggars are very numerous'.[54] Houses of industry were established in each of the counties of Ireland as places of confinement for the sick poor.[55] Their establishment affirmed the principle of state assistance in poverty and medical relief, and the houses of industry, such as the Dublin House of Industry, founded in 1773 at Brunswick Street North, were the precursors of the nineteenth-century workhouses and asylums.

In the nineteenth century, the State's response to the prevailing conditions of poverty, infectious diseases, hunger and destitution was to enact the 'new poor laws'.[56] The Poor Law Amendment Act of 1834 and the Poor Relief (Ireland) Act of 1838 were enacted to deal not with poverty per se, but with 'the detrimental circumstances and dangerous behaviour' that might accompany the condition.[57] The acts were framed by Malthusian thinkers and by political economists who believed that there would remain a perpetual section of the population living below subsistence level, since there was a natural tendency of populations to increase at a rate faster than the means of subsistence.[58] This view gave rise to a system of State assistance that was designed to render poor relief so unattractive as to be a deterrent to population growth, destitution and idleness.[59] The new poor laws shifted the control of the administration of poverty from the local parish to a more centralized form of control, a three-man Poor Law Commission that was empowered to establish union districts or 'unions'; each union was required to establish its own workhouse for the purpose of administering poor relief.[60] A board of guardians, comprising elected local representatives and ex-officio members, administered each workhouse.[61] The paid officers included a master, a matron, a medical officer, a porter and, if directed by the Poor Law Commissioners, a schoolmaster and a schoolmistress.[62]

The new poor laws made clear distinctions between being poor and being destitute and between being able-bodied and being sick. In this way, the new poor laws distinguished between the 'undeserving' and the 'deserving' poor.[63] Since the laws were constructed to reduce state dependency and promote self-reliance, to teach the idle the value of work, and to ensure a form of recompense for charity received, the regime in the workhouse was designed to act as a deterrent for those able-bodied that might otherwise be capable of providing for themselves.[64] George Cornwall Lewis, who was associated with the introduction of the workhouse system into Ireland, declared that the principle of the system was to 'offer everybody relief, but make it so disagreeable that none but those in real want will accept it'.[65] All who entered the workhouse encountered a regime of strict discipline that was designed to ensure their 'due subordination'; at the South Dublin Union, men, women and children of the same families were segregated, received a meagre diet, and the able-bodied among them were put to work in a range of activities that included the care of sick fellow inmates.[66]

By 1851, 163 workhouses with a combined total population of 206,504 had been established in the various poor law union districts.[67] While it was created for the relief of destitution, the Irish workhouse system soon became an important mechanism for medical relief; each workhouse had an infirmary, containing a separate male and female sick ward. Debilitation of inmates, overcrowding and outbreaks of diseases such as cholera and typhus accounted for much of the sickness in the workhouses. In 1854, it was reported that the North Dublin Union had become an institution in which many had 'sought and found its shelter, solely as an hospital'.[68]

This evolution of workhouses into hospitals and the increasing involvement of the Poor Law Commissioners in medical relief in Ireland were attributable to the high incidence of illness that necessitated their adaptation as institutions for the care of the sick.[69] Furthermore, along with their responsibility for administering the Poor Law (Ireland) Act, the Poor Law Commissioners also administered the Medical Charities Act of 1851, which established the local dispensary system.[70] Burke explains that, as the nineteenth century progressed, there occurred a general reduction in pauperism, resulting in greater availability of space in the work-houses, and there was a greater tendency on the part of dispensary doctors to refer acutely ill patients to the workhouse.[71]

The practice of admitting the sick directly into the workhouse became regular-ized through the provisions of the Poor Law Amendment Act of 1862, opening up the workhouse to sick poor who were not destitute and resulting in an increase in the proportion of sick persons relative to other inmates.[72] Of the total work-house population in Ireland, the percentage registered in the workhouse hospitals had risen from 14 per cent in 1851 to 34 per cent in 1872.[73] The workhouses had become de facto 'union hospitals'. During the 1850s and 1860s, the workhouse infirmaries were receiving persons with a variety of medical conditions, including apoplexy, asthma, cancer, consumption, dysentery, gangrene, pleurisy and small-pox.[74] Combined records for the North and South Dublin Unions for the year 1875 indicate that over 30 per cent of residents died in the workhouses in that year.[75]

The Lord Mayor of Cork John Arnott found a depressing scene when he vis-ited the Cork Workhouse in 1859:

> I was shocked, nay, appalled, from my observation of the state of the children … Scrofula has so affected these young creatures that there was scarcely one of them that I examined that did not bear plain and frightful tokens that their blood had been wasted to that degree that ... [it] was only a medium of dis-seminating debility and disease.[76]

At the South Dublin Union, conditions were equally unfavourable for the child inmates, who risked premature death from 'not having vigour to resist the attack of any acute disease'.[77] Mr Henry Price, a Guardian of the South Dublin Union, reported on the serious overcrowding that he found there:

> [The patients] are very much crowded, and in numerous instances patients in the infirmary and hospital wards are sleeping two, and in some instances three, in a bed at this moment.[78]

Dr George B. Owens, a Poor Law Guardian, commented on the condition of the 'able bodied' men in this same workhouse:

> The total number of able-bodied men is 330. They are called able-bodied men; but you would not think them so if you were to see them.[79]

An important principle of the workhouse system was that the pauper was 'bound to give as much labour as his health permits in return for the relief he receives'.[80] On this principle, able-bodied inmates were set to work and, in this way, able-bodied women were required to act as nurses in the workhouse infirmary. These untrained pauper nurses cared for the sick under the supervision of the matron, who herself was untrained in the care of the sick. While a salaried (trained) nurse assisted by the able-bodied female inmates was generally employed in the larger workhouses, pauper nurses alone cared for the sick in the smaller workhouses.[81]

Pauper nurses were selected on the basis of their physical capacity to work and not on the basis of any desire to nurse the sick; they were described as 'selfish and ignorant – deplorably ignorant – utterly devoid of experience, and when an emergency arises are altogether at a loss to know how to act'.[82] In the 1870s, an Irish poor law doctor described the pauper nurses as being 'restrained by no sense of decency or religion, loud voiced, quarrelsome and abusive'.[83] Many were less than capable of caring for the sick in their charge, being frequently in poor health themselves or being old, feeble and illiterate.[84]

Workhouse reform

The reform of the workhouses in England was greatly advanced as a result of lobbying by upper-class social reformers, including Lady Twining and the philanthropist William Rathbone, and by the establishment of the Workhouse Visiting Society.[85] Social reformers pointed to the failings of the workhouse system, which included the inadequate and incompetent nursing. Their concern was part of a broader ideological debate about the functions and dysfunctions of the poor law system. However, the reports of the poor conditions for the inmates in the workhouse infirmaries led to a more immediate concern to ameliorate these same conditions and to bring about a regime of order, where disorder was seen to exist. In Ireland, the efforts to reform the workhouse infirmaries assumed a peculiarly Irish expression, with the Sisters of Mercy playing a key role.

Since pauper nurses were drawn from the poorer class, then the characteristics of their class were also attributable to them; criticism of the poorer class was generally couched in terms that bemoaned their lack of moral character. This lack of moral character was referred to in a report of the Board of Guardians of the Limerick Workhouse in 1860, which noted that 'there appears to be an entire absence of moral control over either nurses or patients'.[86] The solution to this absence of moral control was evident to members of the Limerick Board of Guardians, when it proposed the establishment of 'some central controlling authority' in its workhouse infirmary.[87] The Guardians believed that the employment of nuns from the local convent to act as nurses would provide the necessary skill and the moral qualities essential in a workhouse containing 480 sick persons.

The proposal to initiate the entry of religious sisters into the Limerick workhouse infirmary occurred in an atmosphere of sectarianism.[88] In the face of opposition from Protestant members of the Board and from the Poor Law Commissioners who desired that the workhouse infirmaries should remain non-denominational, the

Roman Catholic members of the Board insisted on appointing three members of the local congregation of the Sisters of Mercy to act as nurses. In its efforts to persuade the Poor Law Commissioners of the benefits that would accrue from employing the sisters, the Board of Guardians declared:

> It is now well understood that the art of nursing is a difficult one to learn, and that it requires, not only great experience, but also considerable intelligence, and for its perfection, the highest moral qualities. The wellbeing of the sick and the cure of disease, depends as much on the combination of these qualities in the nurses as on the skill of the medical officer.[89]

The Sisters of Mercy had thirty years of experience in developing their nursing methods and had successfully taken over the management of the nursing arrangements at the Charitable Infirmary in Dublin in 1854, where they were praised for their disposition of 'disinterested and heroic charity'.[90] The members of the Limerick Board of Guardians were aware of the nuns' achievements as military nurses in the Crimea, and were anxious to procure their services.

The appointment of the first Sisters of Mercy to the Limerick workhouse was secured in 1861. Although answerable to the Master and Matron, the Sisters took partial charge of the workhouse hospital.[91] Within a few short years, the Board of Guardians had lost much of their control over the appointment of nuns as nurses and over the day-to-day running of the workhouse infirmary.[92] This state of affairs was the result of the independent stance taken by the Sisters of Mercy in appointing nuns as nurses without reference to the Board of Guardians and in seeking total control over their own work and that of the trained nurses in the infirmary. While they did not undergo formal nurse training but had developed their skills through instruction from their superiors, the nuns who entered the Limerick workhouse were capable of providing a skilled nursing service, performing a wide range of functions, including dressing wounds, lancing boils, compounding and administering medicines, and managing the diet of the sick.[93]

By 1895, sixty-three boards of guardians had placed their workhouse infirmaries in the hands of nuns, a state of affairs that was partly attributable to the fact that Catholic nationalists had taken over many of the boards of guardians after the 1870s.[94] While the entry of religious sisters into the workhouse hospitals improved conditions for the inmates, by the end of the nineteenth century, the general conditions and the arrangements for medical and surgical treatments remained wholly unsuitable.[95] The low standard of nursing would remain one of the most serious defects of the workhouse hospital. Despite the reforms, pauper nurses were still the norm as late as the 1890s, when there were reports of poor quality of nursing care and the continuing use of workhouse inmates as nurses with complete charge of the patients during night hours. Thus, while the entry of nuns as nurses into the workhouse hospitals represented the principal element of workhouse reform, the reform was only partial when compared with the nursing reforms that had been achieved in the voluntary hospitals by the 1890s.

The fact that Irish nuns controlled and delivered nursing services in the work-house and in some of the voluntary hospitals, despite not having formal professional training, was a testament to their power and authority in Irish society. While they did not concern themselves with the later campaign for state registration, nuns would eventually go on to establish a power base within lay nursing in Ireland.[96]

Aside from the workhouse infirmary, other state services for medical relief for the sick poor included the public dispensary service, the County Infirmaries, the fever hospitals and the lunatic asylums. Introduced under the Medical Charities Act of 1851, the public dispensary service had one or more qualified medical officers and some employed a midwife to attend to poor women in confinement. The dispensaries provided an important and relatively inexpensive system of medical relief for the poor throughout Ireland and continued virtually unchanged until the Health Act of 1970.[97] By the late nineteenth century, the dispensary service had provided a structure around which a home nursing service for the sick poor could develop. This service was provided by a number of voluntary schemes, the most prominent of which were the Queen Victoria's Jubilee Institute for Nurses, and the Lady Dudley Nursing Scheme.[98] Both of these schemes provided a nursing service until the 1950s and were the forerunners of the modern public health nursing service.

The voluntary hospitals and the Dublin School

Along with the workhouse infirmary, the charity or voluntary hospital was the other principal means of providing institutional care for the sick poor. Founded in the eighteenth and early nineteenth centuries on the basis of social need and humanitarian motivation, the voluntary hospitals became an important means of medical relief in the Irish cities that experienced poverty and frequent outbreaks of infectious diseases during the nineteenth century. In these institutions, the conditions of the sick poor and those of their carers became yet another expression of these same social ills.[99]

Boards of governors, acting in a voluntary capacity and comprising wealthy philanthropists, members of the aristocracy and the medical profession, administered the voluntary hospitals. Salaried staff comprised the steward, who had responsibility for overall administration, the apothecary, and the matron, who was responsible for the female staff and for food and linen.[100]

Dublin had a large number of voluntary hospitals, most of which were located in and around the city centre. By the middle of the nineteenth century, a growing population of urban poor, many of whom lived in tenements that were formerly eighteenth-century Georgian town houses, availed of the services of the voluntary hospitals.[101] In the hospital ward, the sick poor experienced a regime of discipline and close surveillance, and were granted food, housing and treatment of disease in return for their contribution to the development of medical science.[102]

At the start of the nineteenth century, the roots of scientific medicine were firmly in place in Ireland. In the Georgian era, the School of Medicine at Trinity

College, the Royal College of Physicians of Ireland, the Royal College of Surgeons in Ireland, and the Apothecaries Hall were founded, as were many of Dublin's principal voluntary hospitals.[103] By the nineteenth century's end, enormous improvements in the treatment and care of persons entering hospital had been achieved through scientific advances that included the identification of pathological bacteria and the introduction of antiseptic surgery and anaesthetics. These improvements were the result of a revolution in scientific medicine that began in France, Austria and Germany and was characterized by the development of new medical and surgical treatments informed by the sciences of experimental physiology and pathological anatomy.[104]

During a fifty-year period after about 1820, when the clinical, diagnostic and teaching methods of the hospitals of Paris and Vienna were introduced, Dublin became a world-renowned centre for medical education.[105] When Queen Victoria's reign began in 1837, Dublin had no less than thirty hospitals and the period following her accession has been described as the 'golden age of Irish medicine'.[106] In this period, the Dublin Medical School flourished and in this renaissance in Irish medicine, a medical elite embraced technological, diagnostic and therapeutic innovations; many became leading international figures in the development of medical science, and their names entered the lexicon of modern medicine.[107] Among the 'galaxy of medical men' associated with the Dublin School were the physicians Robert Graves, William Stokes and Dominic Corrigan, the surgeons James Cusack and Abraham Colles, the anatomist James McCartney, and the eye and ear surgeon William Wilde.[108] These medical men developed new knowledge about the nature of disease and its treatment. For example, Robert Graves replaced the old regime of treating fevers by starving, purging and bleeding with a new regime of care based on feeding the febrile person.[109] Upon his return from continental Europe, Graves also introduced the stethoscope and 'a vast variety of information upon every subject connected with medicine', and he introduced a new system of clinical instruction at the Meath Hospital in 1823.[110] John MacDonnell performed the first operation under general anaesthetic in Ireland at the Richmond Surgical Hospital in 1847 and, by the late nineteenth century, complex invasive surgical operations were the norm in Dublin hospitals.[111]

The association between the Dublin voluntary hospitals and the various medical schools in the city was the necessary condition for the success of the Dublin School, which in 1854 was considered to be 'one of the best schools in Europe for the education of professional youth'.[112] The voluntary hospital became the location for the growth and the reorganization of medical knowledge, and the relationship of clinical observation, teaching and research began to be established.[113] By the middle of the nineteenth century, medical education had established a distinct modus operandi of combining theoretical and clinical instruction, and hospitals that admitted medical students, or 'pupils', were designated as 'clinical hospitals'.

The voluntary hospital became the power base of the medical profession; according to the English doctor Henry Rumsey, the hospital was 'the proper field of *technical* training … where every improvement in subordinate therapeutics is tried under scientific direction'.[114] The reputation of the instructing physician or surgeon enhanced the reputation of the clinical hospital and this reputation acted as an inducement for pupils to attend. The relationship between the clinical hospital and the medical school was thus a decidedly reciprocal one, and the success of medical education depended on the availability of multiple hospital cases to provide the pupil with clinical exemplars of disease.

There was great prestige attached to being designated a 'clinical' hospital, in that it afforded its associated doctors and surgeons an enhanced status and a means of professional advancement. The Dublin Hospitals Commission of 1887 recognized this fact, observing that 'a hospital connexion seems to be almost a *sine qua non* for professional advancement'.[115]

The Medical Act of 1858 established the General Medical Council and with it the registration of medical training and professional regulation of the medical profession in Ireland. The old system of academic medicine based on Greek and Latin texts had been replaced by a system based on empirical science, supported by research and teaching.[116] Scientific medicine emerged as the dominant paradigm in the treatment of disease; the new paradigm was being expressed in a range of activities, including anatomical research, medical and surgical therapeutics, and medical training. The relationship of clinical teaching to medical knowledge was established and so also was the relationship of medical knowledge to the treatment and possible elimination of disease.

Deficiencies in the nursing arrangements

While the 'golden age' of the Dublin School led to rapid developments in medical and surgical treatments, nursing in the voluntary hospitals did not reflect the advances made in the period. Nursing care was provided by untrained nurses, most of whom were uneducated women recruited from the same population of urban poor that availed of the medical relief on offer in the voluntary hospitals.

Having the status of a servant, the nurse performed a specialized form of domestic work, looking after the domestic arrangements of the hospital household, and doing everything that the doctor did not do in relation to the care of the sick.[117] Many nurses were married women with large families and some worked until they were incapacitated from infirmity or old age; such incapacity no doubt curtailed their ability to care effectively for the patients in their charge. Since most nurses received no formal training for their role in the care of the sick, the nursing care was generally of a very poor standard.

While there were efforts in the nineteenth century to bring about improvements in hospital amenities such as lighting, heating, ventilation, water supply, and sanitation, contemporaneous reports bear accounts of frugal living conditions for both patients and their carers; the hospital wards could be cold, dirty and in poor repair.[118] The venereal cases admitted to the Westmorland Lock Hospital in Dublin did not have hospital garments and wore their own clothes when not in bed. The absence of bed screens meant that the privacy of patients was not assured; in evidence to the Select Committee on Dublin Hospitals in 1854, the Senior Surgeon of the Lock Hospital Dr Thomas Byrne remarked:

> [The screens] would not much be wanted: those things entail expense: we are too poor to have superfluities and luxuries.[119]

The Lock Hospital was not unique in not having screens to protect patients' privacy; during the first part of the nineteenth century, maintaining privacy for members of the poorer classes in hospital was generally not seen as necessary.[120]

Nurses often fared little better than their patients. They were housed in living quarters adjacent to the hospital wards, undertook strenuous work for long hours and received poor pay, often in the form of bread and beer or gin, and they were generally required to cook their own food. They lacked adequate sanitary facilities and many had several members of their family housed with them in their accommodation quarters. Insufficient to provide adequate food and clothing, their meagre salary was most likely supplemented with provisions, which they procured from the hospital stock.[121]

The untrained nurse's working conditions were related to the social stratum from which she was drawn. Being recruited from the poorer class, in the public mind, the nurse's work amounted to little more than 'a specialized form of charring'.[122] As well as being a function of her actual social background, the nurse's low social standing was also the result of reports of her behaviour; 'great evils' were associated with the conduct of untrained nurses.[123] There were numerous complaints of ill behaviour and neglect of duty, which frequently resulted in dismissals from service.[124] Reports of drunkenness, thieving from patients and sluttish behaviour were frequently laid before the boards of management of the Dublin hospitals. At Sir Patrick Dun's Hospital in 1835, Nurse Finnamore was dismissed for accepting a gratuity of spirits, while in 1837, two other nurses were dismissed, one for drunkenness and one for violence of temper, and there were other dismissals at the same hospital for insolence, irregularity, neglect of duty, and misconduct.[125] In evidence to the House of Commons Select Committee on Dublin Hospitals in 1854, Dr Thomas Byrne reported that many of the nurses at Dublin's Lock Hospital were dismissed for drunkenness:

> We had to drive out some of them. When I was first there some of them were great drunkards.[126]

At the Dublin House of Industry Hospital in 1871, the Board of Governors considered the cases of Nurses Caldwell, Rutledge and Turner, who were implicated in the pilfering of hospital stock.[127] Later in 1878 at the same hospital, Nurses McEvoy and Bannister were suspended for being under the influence of drink.[128] Misconduct was punishable by a fine or by dismissal.

The reason why these untrained nurses were disposed to act in the ways that they did was first and foremost because they were of their class, and their behaviour reflected the general behaviour of their class.[129] Many had little or no education and they were not bound by the social mores that restricted the upper classes.[130] Their propensity to consume alcohol was not for gratuitous purposes alone, since beer and gin drinking to excess were common in all walks of society; alcohol was considered to have medicinal benefits, and employers frequently dispensed it to workers as a stimulant when extra physical effort was required.[131] Along with its assumed properties as a stimulant, alcohol helped nurses to cope with unpleasant aspects of their work, such as wound smells, and it was believed that alcohol could confer protection against infections, such as typhus, scarlet fever and diphtheria.[132]

The case for reforming hospital nursing

While bad nursing was not the greatest of social evils, it was of such concern that it became an important project for social reformers in the late nineteenth century.[133] The campaign to remove the untrained nurse from hospital and domiciliary nursing began in England in the 1860s and 1870s and this campaign would later be conducted in Dublin in the 1880s. The success of the Dublin School in developing medical science provided the most urgent rationale for reforming hospital nursing. The project of hospital scientific medicine had advanced with such rapidity that the untrained nurse in the voluntary hospital was being rendered incapable of meeting the needs of either the patient or the medical man. Being of the servant class, the hospital nurse had attained a reputation of being uncouth and unreliable and, like her class, was seen as lacking in morals. Scientific medicine needed the assurance that prescribed treatments would be administered accurately and their effects recorded and clearly understood. It required a nurse properly trained in care of the sick and acting under the direction of the medical man, and it required persons who could supervise the nursing care. In the hospital ward and the sick room, scientific medical care needed continuous patient supervision by a competent observer.[134] Robert Graves defined nursing expertise as experience of and familiarity with new medical therapeutics and clinical knowledge of symptomatology.[135] The Dublin surgeon James M. Prior Kennedy believed that good nursing was knowing *when* to summon skilled advice from a surgeon or resident pupil when a serious change in a surgical patient was observed.[136] James Anderson of the London Hospital stressed the vital role of observation in medical cases:

> For the patient the medical nurse should have first an *observant eye* ... The cultivation of the faculty of observation is most important for a nurse, and may, if carefully trained become keener day by day. The observant eye is most necessary in medical cases, which are often very intricate, and where it is not always easy to see what is the matter. Hence a nurse should cultivate the 'clinical instinct' which will enable her to see what is the matter with the patient almost at first sight, and to tell whether the patient is improving or getting worse.[137]

Florence Nightingale also placed emphasis on the faculty of observation in sick nursing:

> The most important practical lesson that can be given to nurses is to teach them what to observe – how to observe – what symptoms indicate improvement – what the reverse – which are of importance – which are of none … For it may safely be said, not that the habit of ready and correct observation will by itself make us useful nurses, but that without it we shall be useless with all our devotion …[138]

This observer role could be expressed only if the nurse was conversant in clinical signs and symptoms, their causes and significance and in the therapeutic and adverse effects of medical treatments. To be a good observer, she should be trustworthy in accurately recording what she observed. She should therefore be an educated woman, capable of receiving instruction in subjects related to scientific medicine and she should be of good moral character.

Conclusions

The new class structures and new relationships between the classes that developed in the wake of the Industrial Revolution came to represent the context for the management of poverty and the provision of charity and medical relief in the nineteenth century. Aside from the workplace, the workhouse infirmary and the voluntary hospital were the principal public arenas where the rich and poor came into close contact with each other, and here the richer class saw at first hand the conditions of poverty, poor sanitation and disease, conditions that were seen to represent the moral poverty of the poor. It was in these institutions that the precursor of the modern nurse was found; she was of the same lower class as the inmates for whom she cared and her attributes as a member of her class, along with her actual behaviour in nursing the sick, meant that she too was considered to be morally poor.

In the voluntary hospital the upper class could direct the lower class onto a more moral path and, in this regard, the untrained nurse as much as the patient was a target of moral improvement.[139] Through her work and through her good example, a nurse of better moral character could be a transmitter of upper-class values of order and good living. A nurse of 'exemplary conduct and character' would be better placed to treat the illnesses that were held to be the result of immoral conduct.[140] To be this purveyor of upper-class values and to be a skilled medical auxiliary, the nurse should be recruited from a 'better class' of persons. As early as 1854, this new nurse was envisioned by Mary Stanley, a friend of Nightingale, who declared that the nurse of the future belonged to 'a class of persons which remains to be created'.[141]

2 'Nursing arrangements'

Nursing policy in Dublin in the late nineteenth century

The voluntary hospitals were funded from central and local government and from charitable fundraising. The bodies that controlled the funds of the hospitals wielded considerable influence in hospital management policy, including nursing policy. These bodies included the Dublin Hospital Sunday Fund, an influential fundraising movement representing upper class views on social policy in the domain of the voluntary hospitals, and the Dublin Hospitals Commission, a parliamentary commission set up in 1885 to examine the management of the Dublin hospitals in receipt of the annual Parliamentary grant. In the 1870s and 1880s, both of these bodies conducted extensive inquiries into the management of the principal Dublin hospitals, including inquiries into their nursing arrangements. The reports of these inquiries highlighted major deficiencies in the nursing arrangements in those hospitals staffed by untrained nurses and each contained explicit policy statements on nursing.[1] Setting down a clear agenda for the reform of hospital nursing, the reports were highly influential in determining the conduct of subsequent nursing policy, including policy on nurse training.

The Dublin Hospital Sunday Fund

The Dublin Hospital Sunday Fund (DHSF) was founded in 1874 as a fundraising movement for the hospitals of Dublin. Its membership represented powerful and influential interests in social policy in late nineteenth-century Dublin. Its patron was the Lord Lieutenant, its President was the Earl of Meath, and its Executive Council included the President of the King's and Queen's Colleges of Physicians, the President of the Royal College of Surgeons in Ireland, members of the Dublin Anglo-Irish aristocracy, professionals and businessmen, medical men, and Anglican clergymen.[2]

The Fund's method of fundraising was an annual church collection conducted on a single designated Sunday of each year during church services in participating parishes. At the time of its founding, it was envisaged that the Fund would be a national scheme, embracing the Catholic and Protestant churches. However, while the scheme received the support of Archbishop Trench, the Protestant Archbishop of Dublin, it did not receive the support of his Roman Catholic counterpart. Archbishop Cullen rejected the centralization of fundraising, arguing that the proposed scheme was not the best way to attract donations.[3] In its first annual report for the year 1874, the Executive Council of the DHSF reported that the authorities of the Roman Catholic Church and the principal Roman Catholic hospitals refused to 'have anything to do with the movement'.[4] The Council noted that it was 'with great regret' that it had passed a resolution to the effect that the Mater Misericordiae Hospital and St Vincent's Hospital could not be included in the list of hospitals that were to receive a share of the annual collection made by the Fund.

The non-participation of the official Roman Catholic Church was at variance with the experience of similar fundraising movements in England, such as those in Manchester, Salford, London, Birmingham and Liverpool, in which cases the Council of the Dublin movement observed, 'all denominations, without exception, co-operated'.[5] However, Dublin was unlike any of the aforementioned English cities. In Dublin, where religious differences could be pronounced, there was a prevailing undercurrent of sectarian mistrust; Catholic suspicion of proselytizing by Anglicans may have underlain the decision of the Catholic hierarchy not to participate in the movement. When asked by the House of Commons Select Committee on Dublin Hospitals of 1854 whether religious differences had anything to do with the difficulty in obtaining subscriptions for Dublin's hospitals, Dr Dominic Corrigan of the Dublin House of Industry Hospitals remarked that 'religious differences have to do with everything in Ireland'.[6] By participating in the DHSF movement, the Roman Catholic hospitals would be in receipt of monies that were, in effect, donated by non-Catholics. For Catholics, this would effectively amount to 'taking the soup', a position that would be unsatisfactory for a Catholic hierarchy that was asserting its independence in a period of growing nationalist consciousness.

Committee on Nursing

As a fundraising movement, the DHSF was a success and the benefits accruing for the Fund's participating hospitals were evident after the first year of its operation.[7] In its report for the year 1875, the Council of the DHSF expressed itself satisfied with 'the continued and increased success of the movement'. From the outset, it was clear that it was the wish of the Fund that the monies that it donated to its participating hospitals should be put to improving the management of the hospitals:

> The Council rejoice that efforts of the ... [Fund] have thus exercised a beneficial effect on the management of Dublin Hospitals in addition to the benefits conferred on them by the increase to their funds.[8]

The Council encouraged its participating hospitals to continue their efforts at improving their management:

> The Council do not wish to particularize any Hospitals, but trust that the good sense of their Managers will lead them to continue the improvements in

administration which seem to have been the direct result of their connexion to the Hospital Sunday Fund.[9]

Throughout its early years, the DHSF was generating sums of £4000 a year for distribution to the Dublin hospitals. In 1878, the Council of the Fund reasoned that, since it was providing such large sums of money to its participating hospitals, it was 'bound to have regard to the efficiency of the arrangements for the care of the patients in these institutions'. At a meeting held on 22 October 1878, the Council adopted the following resolution:

> That a Committee be appointed … to inquire into the arrangements for Nursing in each of the Hospitals participating in the Hospital Sunday Fund, and to report to a future meeting of the Council.[10]

The Committee on Nursing was constituted with a membership of eleven that included the Fund's President and Vice-President, its Honorary Secretaries, T. Pim Junior, T. W. Grimshaw, and R. O'B Furlong, the Dean of the Chapel Royal, doctors Evory, Kennedy and Duffey, and Messers D. Drummond and A. Shackleton.[11] In the course of its inquiries, the Committee on Nursing visited fourteen Dublin hospitals and, following three months of 'careful investigation', the Committee presented its *Report on the Nursing Arrangements in the Dublin Hospitals*, 'a valuable and detailed report', which the Executive Council of the DHSF adopted on 22 January 1879.[12] The report contained a summary of the Committee's findings in respect of 'defects' that it had identified in the nursing arrangements in the hospitals visited. The report also contained 'observations and recommendations'.

The Committee on Nursing reported that in seven of the fourteen hospitals visited, the nursing arrangements were 'under the control of persons who have never had any special training for their duties'. The seven hospitals were the City of Dublin Hospital, Dr Steevens' Hospital, the Meath Hospital, Mercer's Hospital, the Whitworth Hospital, the Adelaide Hospital, and the Dublin Orthopaedic Hospital. At only three hospitals, Sir Patrick Dun's, St Mark's and Cork Street, were the nurses 'directly controlled' by a trained superintendent. At the National Eye and Ear Infirmary and at Rathdown Hospital, 'partial supervision' of nurses was found, while at the Rotunda and Coombe hospitals, only the lying-in nurses were supervised. The Committee also reported that, with the exception of the lying-in departments of the Rotunda and Coombe hospitals, in none of the hospitals was any previous training 'a necessary condition for appointment as [a] nurse'.

In the matter of arrangements for the systematic training of nurses, the Committee on Nursing reported that 'regular schools for the training of nurses as midwives' existed in the lying-in hospitals and at the maternity section of Sir Patrick Dun's Hospital. With the exception of the training arrangements at Sir Patrick Dun's, which was connected with the Dublin Nurses Training Institution at Holles Street, there were 'no establishments for the systematic training of nurses annexed to any of the Hospitals'. While there was 'an arrangement' for probationers at the Adelaide Hospital, the Committee reported that there did not seem to be 'any systematic training carried out at that Hospital'.

The Committee on Nursing observed that the organization of nursing in the various hospital departments was partly dependent on the construction of the hospitals, and it noted that hospitals were 'as a rule badly planned for nursing purposes.' In this connection, the Committee pointed to the enormous variance that existed in the grouping of hospital wards for nursing purposes. For example, at Sir Patrick Dun's Hospital, fifteen wards were organized in four groups, while at the Meath Hospital there were twenty wards in four groups. This variance was a function of the differences both in the size of individual wards and in the numbers of nurses and attendants employed to staff them:

> This arrangement into nursing divisions or groups is in principle correct, but the organization of the divisions is in most cases faulty, either from defective construction of the buildings or from the paucity of attendants.[13]

It appears that a deficiency in one factor could be offset by an improvement in another. At Sir Patrick Dun's Hospital, for example, the problem of the large number of small wards was 'counteracted by the distribution of probationers to each ward'.

The Committee on Nursing also reported on the classification of nurses, or the 'methods in existence for the attendance of the patients'. In many of the large hospitals, each division or ward grouping had a nurse or a head nurse supported by one or two assistant nurses, night nurses and wardmaids. In all of the hospitals, extra nurses were employed for 'special cases'. At Sir Patrick Dun's and the Adelaide hospitals, probationers assisted the nurse. The Committee expressed concern at the insufficient supply of night nurses and the lack of clear definitions of the duties of the ward attendants, assistant nurses and wardmaids. A particular concern was the custom in Dublin hospitals of combining the duties of assistant nurse and wardmaid:

> This is a very serious defect, as persons engaged in scrubbing, removing refuse and other housemaids' duties, cannot be in a fit condition to tend patients, must frequently leave the wards at irregular intervals, and must be drawn from a lower social class than that from which nurses should be derived.[14]

The Committee reported on 'the want of proper codes of printed rules' for nurses, and on defects in the wages, board, lodging and clothing of nurses and assistant nurses. It noted that the term 'assistant nurse' was generally used to denote a bona fide nurse acting as assistant to the head nurse and expecting to become a head nurse in the future. The average wage of a nurse was £13 per annum, while that of an assistant nurse was £8 per annum. The Committee determined that there was a link between nurses' conditions of employment and the recruitment of desirable persons as nurses:

It is quite impossible to expect to get nurses with any degree of training, or of an educated class *without* training, on such low wages, such being the wages of the most ordinary domestic servants. Interviews with the nurses at the hospitals showed that, with few exceptions, the women were below the class of ordinary domestic servants. At Cork-street Hospital, where the wages have been increased, some trained nurses have been obtained, and the nurses are of a higher class than are usually met with elsewhere.[15]

Nurses' sleeping arrangements were also reported to be defective, while the quality of the eating and cooking arrangements varied greatly across the Dublin hospitals. Arrangements for nurses' rest and relaxation were also found to be seriously deficient:

In all the general hospitals, the nurses seem to be over-worked, partly from defective method, and partly from want of sufficient relaxation, air and exercise. The plan which prevails of giving a few hours in the afternoon and evening, once or twice a week, does not suffice to maintain the nurses in proper health.[16]

The Committee sought to establish a link between the state of the nursing arrangements and the general financial state of the Dublin hospitals:

A great deal of the poverty of the Dublin Hospitals arises from the fact that their resources are wasted by there being a much greater number of hospitals in Dublin than is necessary.[17]

This fact represented 'one of the chief difficulties in providing skilled supervision of nursing, and proper training establishments for nurses', and because of their size, few Dublin hospitals could 'afford a sufficient field for the practical training of a reasonable number of probationers'. As a way of addressing these shortcomings, the Committee advised that the smaller hospitals should group or amalgamate. The Committee cited Sir Patrick Dun's Hospital, the National Eye and Ear Infirmary, and the Rathdown Hospital as examples of institutions which had an organized system of trained nurses. On the grounds that most of the hospitals were too small to have 'regular training schools' attached, the Committee proposed the establishment of a centralized training school for the Dublin hospitals:

the Committee suggest that a central home and training institution for nurses be established, where probationers could reside, and receive systematic teaching on subjects collateral to nursing. The probationers from such a home should be sent in detachments to the various hospitals, and there be taught by properly-trained Superintendents of nurses.[18]

It was the Committee's view that the defects in nursing could be remedied through 'organic alterations' in hospital structure and the establishment of nursing divisions in each hospital, and by ensuring that the person in control of nurses should understand nursing and should therefore be a trained nurse. Each nursing division should contain a single head nurse, the proper number of assistant nurses for day and night, and a wardmaid to do housemaid's work. Nurses undertaking probationership training should act in the role of assistant nurses. The practice of employing extra nurses for special cases was considered to be inordinately costly, and it was the Committee's view that extra nurses 'should seldom be required in properly organized institutions'.

The Committee on Nursing set down two principles relating to the locus of responsibility for the training of nurses and the conditions of employment for nurses in training that would remain as central tenets of nursing policy for over a century afterwards:

> The Committee are of the opinion that it is not only the duty of the hospital authorities to provide for the efficient supervision and organization of their nurses … but also that it is their duty to take their part in training nurses, just as it is to train Medical Practitioners.[19]

Hospital authorities were also responsible for the proper care of nurses in training, and conditions of employment were related to recruitment and retention of nurses and, by inference, to the quality of the nursing:

> Until the nurses are better paid, more comfortably lodged and fed, better superintended, and not so overworked as they are at present, it cannot be expected that a better class of nurse will be obtainable, or that respectable women will go to the labour and expense (and personal risk often) of being systematically and carefully trained. The prospects held out for a nurse in a Dublin hospital are usually much less than those in domestic service. In addition to comfortable board, lodging, and uniform, nurses should be paid liberally. They should have regular hours for work, rest and relaxation; and a certain annual holiday of not less than a month.[20]

In its report, the Committee on Nursing made a total of twelve recommendations concerning the nursing arrangements in its participating hospitals, and it advised that each hospital receiving aid from the Fund should comply with its recommendations. The Committee recommended that hospital buildings should be arranged into suitable divisions for nursing purposes. Each hospital should employ a lady superintendent, 'fully capable of carrying out hospital nursing in all its details, and of giving systematic instruction to those who may be placed under her'. Head nurses and assistant nurses should be properly qualified, assistant nurses should not undertake the duties of wardmaids, and the duties of all grades should be defined by printed rules. Nurses should be provided with better accommodation for sleeping and dieting, and better pay, and they should be granted daily relaxation and periodic holidays. Nurses should not cook patients' meals and a 'printed placard' should be displayed, informing patients that nurses who

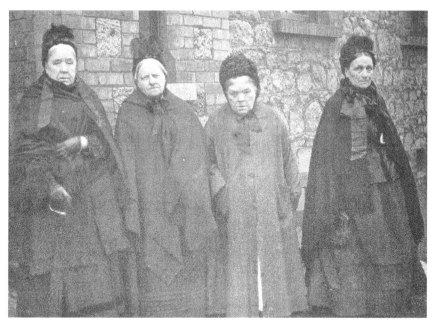

Figure 2.1 Nurses, Meath Hospital, Dublin, 1872

solicited or received money from patients would be subject to instant dismissal. On the training of nurses, the Committee made the single recommendation that every hospital 'should take its part in the training of nurses, either by having a training establishment of its own or by co-operating with other hospitals through a central training establishment'.

In closing its report, the Committee expressed the view that the authorities of all the hospitals should 'do their best, if heartily sustained by public support, to carry out any recommendations, which may be adopted by the Council [of the Fund]'. It expressed confidence that such a response on the part of hospital authorities would result in 'great good … not only for the sick poor, but also to their wealthier neighbours who at present suffer much from the scarcity of good and efficiently trained nurses'.

Influence of the Fund on nursing policy

The Council of the Dublin Hospital Sunday Fund forwarded copies of the report of the Committee on Nursing to all the hospitals participating in the Fund. Hospitals were urged to 'pay special attention to the recommendations at the end of the Report' and were advised that 'any remarks the Managers of your Hospital may favour us with, will meet with best consideration of the Committee'.[21] In replies sent to the Committee, a number of hospitals indicated that they had acted upon the Committee's recommendations. The authorities at the Rotunda

Hospital had endeavoured to carry out the recommendations by preparing a code of rules for nurses and by establishing 'a graduated scale of increased wages, as an encouragement to efficient nursing'. The City of Dublin Hospital replied that many of the Committee's recommendations had 'for some time been acted upon' and it had provided increased accommodation for the nurses by converting one of the wards into a nurses' bedroom. Mercer's Hospital advised the Committee that it was in a position to provide accommodation for a superintendent of nurses, as well as increased accommodation for nurses. Dr Steevens' Hospital reported that the recommendations of the Committee had been adopted; a trained superintendent of nurses was appointed and the nursing arrangements were now complete. The Meath Hospital had the suggestions of the Committee 'under careful consideration'. The authorities of the Adelaide Hospital had 'taken steps to improve the nursing arrangements, and [had] adopted a code of rules for the nursing organization of the Hospital'. These rules provided for the employment of a lady superintendent and four divisional lady nurses, and the Hospital had sent its Lady Superintendent Miss Reynolds to St Bartholomew's Hospital in London for a course in nurse training and hospital management.[22]

In the light of the various responses it received from the participating hospitals, the Committee on Nursing was in a position to report:

> On a review of the information in possession of the Committee, they have much pleasure in observing that the recommendations of the Council have been favourably received, and have already produced beneficial results.[23]

The *Report on the Nursing Arrangements in the Dublin Hospitals* highlighted major defects in the nursing systems of the Dublin hospitals participating in the DHSF movement. The general tone of the report was one of displeasure, and its publication had an immediate and powerful influence on management policy in the hospitals. The Committee on Nursing was quick to establish a link between the awards made by the Fund and the agenda for the reform of hospital nursing, which it had so explicitly established in its report:

> The most substantial difficulty which exists in the way of nursing reform, as of other reforms in the Dublin Hospitals, is financial. All the Dublin Hospitals are poor, but as they are now much richer than they were, owing to the aid afforded by the Hospital Sunday Fund, the contributors and promoters of the fund may justly expect that some of the newly acquired resources may be applied to such reforms as the managers of the fund may suggest.[24]

The DHSF Committee of Distribution had responsibility for the allocation of monies awarded by the Fund, and in its report the Committee on Nursing included the following recommendation:

> The Committee [on Nursing] recommend that in the distribution of the fund in future years, the Committee of Distribution should be instructed that

when making their awards, they should take into consideration the efficiency of the nursing arrangements in the participating institution, and modify the grants accordingly.[25]

The control of monies could act as a powerful weapon in the pursuit of policy goals; the DHSF had relatively large sums of money at its disposal and, according to its rules, it had the prerogative to determine the size of the annual grant that each hospital could receive. Since the findings of the Report of the Committee on Nursing were made public, hospitals felt obliged to reform, and at the same time, were drawn to the additional monies that the Fund could provide.[26]

In allocating funds for the year 1880, the Fund's Committee of Distribution was obliged to consider 'how far those Institutions had carried out the suggestions of the Nursing Committee'.[27] To this end, the Committee of Distribution requested that each hospital should include in its annual returns detailed information on its nursing arrangements, to include information on the structure of the nursing division and the nurses' conditions of employment. It should indicate whether it employed a trained superintendent of nurses and whether the nurses or assistant nurses undertook the duties of wardmaids. Each hospital should provide information on the nurses' dining and sleeping arrangements, and the arrangements for the systematic training of probationers.

On the basis of the information received from participating hospitals, the Committee of Distribution was in a position 'to form a correct estimate of the progress made by ... Institutions, in improving their nursing arrangements'. The Committee was willing to act upon the information received. In its Annual Report of 1880, the Committee of Distribution expressed satisfaction that the participating hospitals had either carried out the recommendations of the Council 'to the fullest extent' or had effected 'partial improvements' in their nursing arrangements. In the case of three hospitals, the Adelaide, the Meath and St Mark's, from which 'sufficient explicit replies' were not received, the Committee of Distribution requested representatives of their respective governing authorities to attend a meeting of the Committee on 12 November 1880 to discuss matters requiring explanation. The Adelaide and St Mark's hospitals satisfied the Committee that they were responding positively to the recommendations of the Committee of Nursing, and it was decided on that basis that they were entitled to receive 'the full proportion' of the Fund. The Committee of Distribution was dissatisfied with the response of the Meath Hospital and, while it refrained from reducing the grant to that Hospital for that year, it resolved 'that a more stringent course should be adopted in future'.[28] This admonishment drew a quick response, and the Medical Board of the Meath Hospital immediately sought the replacement of the untrained Matron Mrs Jones with a trained lady superintendent.[29] The governors of the Meath Hospital initially resisted replacing Mrs Jones, on account of her great capacity for fundraising. However, the governors eventually appointed Miss Elinor Lyons as Lady Superintendent with responsibility to train and supervise the nurses, and they entered into an arrangement for the training of probationers with the Red Cross Nursing Sisters at Harcourt Street.

In its report for the year 1882, the Committee of Distribution reasoned that 'sufficient time had now elapsed to enable the Authorities of the Dublin Hospitals to take steps to remedy the defects in their Nursing Systems'.[30] On this basis, the Committee of Distribution set aside additional monies to distribute to those hospitals that had complied with the recommendations of the Committee on Nursing. Of the fifteen hospitals in receipt of the Fund's annual grant for that year, ten received a bonus payment of 5 per cent for effecting improvements in their nursing arrangements, while the bonus was withheld from the remainder. Through successive years up to and including 1887, the Committee of Distribution continued to exercise its prerogative in awarding or withholding the bonus payment and, in this way, it assumed the role of watchdog of standards.[31]

The DHSF was a significant contributor to the finances of the Dublin hospitals, which were, as a rule, financially not well off in the nineteenth century.[32] The Dublin Hospitals Commission recognized the role of the Fund in bringing about nursing reform when it issued its report in 1887. Referring to the nursing arrangements at the City of Dublin Hospital, the Commission stressed the benefits for hospitals in being associated with the DHSF:

> the nursing arrangements in this hospital ... afford a striking example of the advantages which are capable of being derived from the inspections of hospitals by such a body as the Committee of the Hospital Sunday Fund, and from the system upon which contributions from such a fund are assessed. In the case of the City of Dublin Hospital, the adoption by the Board of the present system of nursing was no doubt influenced by their desire to obtain a larger share in the distribution of that fund by effecting improvements in that branch of their administration in which they had been found deficient.[33]

The members of the Council of the DHSF comprised influential figures in Irish public life and the new nursing arrangements that were put in place on the recommendations of the Fund's Committee on Nursing were in keeping with the views and values of this constituency.[34] Less than a decade after the publication of the report of the Committee on Nursing, enormous changes had taken place in the nursing arrangements in the Dublin hospitals. In its annual report of 1888, the Fund noted that due to 'the efforts of the Council [of the DHSF] to enforce proper nursing arrangements in the Hospitals receiving aid from the Fund' there were no reports of 'defective nursing organization'; the principal recommendations of the Committee on Nursing were now in place:

> Nursing by trained nurses under the inspection of trained Lady Superintendents is now carried out in every Hospital receiving aid from the Fund.[35]

Records indicate that the DHSF continued to operate until 1931.[36] By that year, through its Visiting Committee, the Fund concerned itself more with hospital household and sanitary arrangements and less with the nursing arrangements. In its final year, the grants awarded by the Fund to its participating hospitals were, in relative terms, a much smaller proportion of the hospitals' overall budgets than in its first decade. The Fund's influence on nursing policy had long been overtaken by events, most especially the attainment of state registration in 1919, and by the new and more centralized source of funding available from monies generated by the Irish Hospitals Sweepstakes.[37]

Nursing arrangements and the Dublin Hospitals Commission

Throughout the nineteenth century, a series of statutory commissions was established to inquire into institutions in Dublin that were in receipt of monies from Parliament. These included commissions of inquiry in 1808, 1829 and 1842, a House of Commons Select Committee in 1854, and the Dublin Hospital Inquiry Commission (the South Commission) in 1856. Since these various commissions of inquiry were more concerned with the suitability of the Dublin hospitals as institutions for the instruction of medical pupils, they contained little information on the hospitals' nursing arrangements. Referring to the nursing arrangements at the Westmorland Lock Hospital, the South Commission considered it to be 'of the highest importance that the Matron and the Nurses should be carefully selected with regard to their intelligence and moral character'.[38]

In 1885, the Lord Lieutenant of Ireland Lord Spencer appointed the Dublin Hospitals Commission to 'make an inquiry into the management and working of several hospitals in the City of Dublin'.[39] This Commission was charged with ascertaining whether, in respect of those hospitals receiving annual grants from public funds, the conditions upon which grants were made were being observed and complied with. The Commission examined aspects of hospital management, including the methods of appointing officers, the composition of the boards of governors, the arrangements for medical training, and the possibility of amalgamations between hospitals. The Commission also made extensive inquiries into the hospitals' nursing arrangements. The Dublin Hospitals Commission sat in the Privy Council Chamber at Dublin Castle, was chaired by Sir Rowland Blennerhassett, and published its report on 4 April 1887.[40]

Published less than a decade after the DHSF had forwarded copies of its Committee on Nursing report to the Fund's participating hospitals, the report of the Dublin Hospitals Commission contained evidence concerning the nursing arrangements in the principal Dublin hospitals, and it included specific recommendations concerning hospital nursing. The report provided a clear picture of the nursing arrangements in many of the Dublin hospitals at a time when the movement for the reform of hospital nursing was well advanced.

The Dublin Hospitals Commission reported on the 'circumstances' of fifteen Dublin hospitals, including the major voluntary hospitals and the principal lying-in hospitals in the city.[41] The Commission inquired into the arrangements for nurse training. While training schemes had been instituted in many of the Dublin hospitals, some institutions did not have formal arrangements for the training of nurses and they continued to employ untrained nurses. Evidence taken by the

Commission indicated that the Dublin House of Industry Hospitals and the two principal Catholic-run hospitals in receipt of the Parliamentary grant, the Mater Misericordiae Hospital and the Charitable Infirmary, had not instituted nursing reforms of the kind that were introduced in the Protestant hospitals following the DHSF Committee on Nursing report.

In its report, the Dublin Hospitals Commission referred to the nursing arrangements at the Mater Misericordiae Hospital, which was under the control of the Sisters of Mercy. Thirteen of the sisters at the hospital attended the sick and were assisted by wardmaids. The average attendance was one sister to thirteen beds on day duty and there were six lay night nurses under the charge of the sisters. When 'serious cases' arose during the night, the sister on duty and the house surgeon were summoned. In evidence to the Commission, Dr Christopher J. Nixon, the Senior Physician at the hospital, described the nursing arrangements whereby the nurses were drawn from the 'most intelligent of ward maids' and trained by the sisters, who were not themselves trained nurses.[42] In 'cases of delirium or special urgent cases', additional nurses were employed. When asked as to the nature of instruction required for taking up a position of nurse at the Mater Misericordiae Hospital, Dr Nixon conceded that there was no special provision for the training of nurses. He observed that appointment as a nurse was based upon the aptitude of the sister for her work and he remarked that 'as it is a labour of love they fall into the business of nursing very quickly.' In evidence, Dr Thomas More Madden, a surgeon at the hospital, observed that the 'kindly care and constant attention' proffered by the Sisters of Mercy were very necessary to the care and recovery of women undergoing major gynaecological surgery at the hospital.[43] Notwithstanding the reports of the good quality of the nursing care provided by the sisters, in its report the Commission made explicit reference to the fact that untrained nurses were providing the nursing care at the Mater Misericordiae Hospital.

At the Charitable Infirmary Jervis Street, the Sisters of Mercy were also in charge of the nursing arrangements, but of no other part of hospital administration. Like the situation that obtained at the Mater Misericordiae Hospital, the sisters at the Charitable Infirmary were not 'regularly trained' nurses. According to evidence given by one of the hospital's surgeons, Mr Arthur Chance, the Sisters of Mercy did their duty admirably and it seems that, while they might have lacked formal training, their presence in the hospital was important to the overall management of the institution. Mr Chance observed:

> There are details of nursing that … [the sisters] might learn with advantage, but, on the whole, any shortcomings in this respect are more than counterbalanced by the great and special advantage of their presence in a hospital like Jervis-street. They bring to their task a devotion which it is impossible to hire, and, most important of all, is the immense gain to discipline and moral tone resulting from their presence in the hospital.[44]

Mr Chance went on to state that the sisters looked after the patients very closely, never shirked unpleasant tasks in the conduct of their work, and did not allow 'any mock modesty to interfere with their duty'. He observed that, as long as they remained their best, the public could be assured that the sisters' tenure of office was secure. Mr Edward Thomas Stapleton, a member of the Board of Governors of the Charitable Infirmary, bemoaned the fact that trained nurses were hard to come by in Dublin city, and he was aware that nurses properly trained in hospitals in Liverpool and Birkenhead seemed to thoroughly understand the business of nursing.[45] Mr Stapleton was keen to see the establishment of nurse training at the Charitable Infirmary.

While the nursing care proffered by the Sisters of Mercy at the Charitable Infirmary produced 'economy in management, with increased comfort to the patients', in its report the Dublin Hospitals Commission pointed out that the sisters were not themselves trained nurses. The Commission regarded the nursing arrangements at the hospital as being 'not satisfactory', and it recommended that, since the sisters did not undertake night duty and in view of 'the number and nature of accident cases received', the nurses at the hospital should be carefully trained.

While the Sisters of Mercy were to the forefront in pioneering new methods of nursing in Dublin in the 1830s and later as military nurses in the Crimea, it appears that they were equivocal about the movement for nursing reform that had taken place elsewhere in Dublin. The reasons why the Sisters of Mercy and the Irish Sisters of Charity at St Vincent's Hospital were among the last to introduce nursing reform into their hospitals were related to a number of factors. Since the Catholic hospitals were not participants in the DHSF movement, they did not come under the sphere of influence of the Fund, and were not directly affected by the imperative to reform hospital nursing that had existed in the wake of the DHSF's Committee on Nursing report. By the late 1880s, the Sisters of Mercy had a well-developed system of sick nursing that had greatly improved the care of hospitalized persons.[46] For the sisters at the Mater Misericordiae Hospital and the Charitable Infirmary, the work of sick nursing was held to be an integral part of what it was to *be* a Sister of Mercy; sick nursing required a disposition that could not be derived from systematic training alone. In their role in Irish education in the period, nuns believed that excellence in teaching was a product of devotion, care and good basic education, rather than technical training.[47] Similarly, in their involvement in sick nursing and hospital management, their approach was to resist technical-professional training. Fahey refers to this disposition as an 'anti-technical attitude, [by which] nuns introduced progress through diligence, care and order in daily routines, rather than through the development and acquisition of formal professional skills'.[48] Their resistance to technical training was also related to their considerable corporate knowledge, which they developed from their extensive experience of nursing the sick poor in their own homes.[49]

However, as far as the Dublin Hospitals Commission was concerned, the Catholic hospitals were decidedly 'outside the Pale', inasmuch as they had failed to become involved in the movement for nursing reform; they continued to employ untrained nurses in their hospital wards and they failed to introduce arrangements for the proper training of nurses. The finger of officialdom was now firmly pointing in their direction.

In its report, the Commission expressed admiration for those hospitals that had introduced formal arrangements for the training of nurses, such as Sir Patrick Dun's Hospital and the City of Dublin Hospital. Sir Patrick Dun's Hospital had appointed a trained lady superintendent of nurses for the purpose of providing private nurses for extern service, and the Commission noted that this 'experiment' had been 'attended with marked success'.[50] The Commission also praised the high quality of the midwifery service provided by Sir Patrick Dun's midwifery department, which it attributed to the six-month course of training provided for the maternity nurses attending the lying-in women. In evidence to the Commission, the Reverend Dr Samuel Haughton, a member of the Board of Governors of Sir Patrick Dun's, noted that the hospital was the first in Dublin to introduce a system of trained nurses, having appointed a 'properly trained' lady superintendent as long ago as 1867. The hospital trained private nurses whose extern duties could realise £300 per annum for the hospital, and it had a complement of three staff nurses, one night superintendent, and eighteen probationers. This represented a ratio of one nurse to five and three-quarter beds on day duty, and one nurse to eleven and a half beds on night duty. The hospital attached 'extreme importance' to night nurses, believing that they should be 'the most proficient, the most active, and the most intelligent women in the house'. Reverend Haughton remarked that 'the day for turning on an old woman to attend seventy beds has long passed by' and he described the hospital's policy on nurses' age:

> With regard to the ages of our nurses, we won't take them under twenty-five and we ask them to provide for themselves elsewhere on reaching forty-five. When a woman in an hospital comes to the age of fifty years she had better look out for a quieter berth.[51]

Sir Patrick Dun's Hospital also believed in adequate and proper remuneration for nurses; the hospital paid a salary of between £20 and £30 per annum, as compared with £12 in other hospitals. Its extern nurses earned £27 per annum. Reverend Haughton expressed surprise in having read other evidence to the Commission as to the 'extreme excellence of the nursing system in all the Dublin hospitals', given the low salaries on offer. He remarked:

> I rubbed my eyes and said that was all nonsense. If a man asks me to dine with him, and gives me a bottle of Gladstonian claret, and tells me it is Lafitte, I won't drink it. You cannot get nurses whose services are worth £26 a year at £12.[52]

The nursing arrangements at the City of Dublin Hospital were also the subject of praise by the Commission. The hospital had made 'admirable' improvements in its system of nursing, in response to deficiencies pointed out by the DHSF Committee on Nursing. In evidence, Mr H. Gray Croly, a surgeon at the City of Dublin Hospital, described the nursing system at the hospital as being 'admirably done', with a lady superintendent employed on a salary of £100 per annum and probationership training in place since the City of Dublin Nursing Institution opened in 1883.[53] According to Mr Croly, the probationers from the Institution learned their work and did it well. Mr deCourcy Wheeler, a director of the Institution, gave evidence that the Institution was in its infancy and that, in consequence, nurses were employed at the hospital from all the 'highest schools of training' in Liverpool, Manchester and London.[54] The City of Dublin Hospital made no distinction between day and night nurses, the entire corps of nurses taking day and night duty in rotation. Mr Croly believed that 'a most skilled and trustworthy nurse should be in charge of night duty'.

The Dublin Hospitals Commission reported that the nursing arrangements at the Meath Hospital had been previously 'very defective', but that they had greatly improved in recent years. The nursing arrangements were under the control of a lady superintendent, who was highly qualified, having trained in hospitals in Liverpool and Cork, attended lectures given by a medical man, and received instruction in the management of the sick bed. Mercer's Hospital employed a lady superintendent, five nurses, three attendants, and two night nurses. The system of nursing worked most satisfactorily and the nurses were found to be 'at all times most attentive to their duties and kind to the patients'.[55] The Senior Surgeon to Mercer's Hospital Mr Edward Stamer O'Grady gave evidence that the day nurses were 'as a rule, extremely good – some of them … the best in Dublin.'[56] He reported that the night nurses were in the past 'atrociously wretched', but that the hospital had recently appointed a new night nurse, 'a most excellent woman of good character and with a diploma'. Cork Street Fever Hospital had a lady superintendent, a 'most capable officer' who, with the approval of the Board, could appoint and dismiss the nurses.[57]

The Commission heard conflicting evidence concerning the nursing arrangements at the Dublin House of Industry Hospitals (Richmond, Hardwicke and Whitworth Hospitals). Some of the hospital's representatives, including the surgeons William Stokes, James M. Prior Kennedy and William Thompson, gave evidence of defective nursing arrangements in the Richmond Surgical Hospital.[58] Stokes reported that there was no trained superintendent of nurses 'in the modern acceptance of the term', while Kennedy reported instances of 'inefficiency' and drunkenness. In evidence, other members of the Board of Governors, including physicians and lay members, gave positive reports on the nursing arrangements in the Whitworth Medical and Hardwicke Fever hospitals. The physician Dr Samuel Gordon expressed the opinion that the nursing at the Whitworth was very fair and that the nursing at the Hardwicke could not be surpassed.

The Commission also took evidence concerning the arrangements for the training of nurses as midwives at the city's principal lying-in hospitals. In evidence, the Master of the Rotunda expressed himself satisfied with the hospital's nursing arrangements, where as many as thirty nurses had obtained diplomas in midwifery in some years, but he expressed concern that while the head nurse was well acquainted with the system, she should be a lady trained in general nursing. As this was not the case, he believed that a lady trained in general nursing could instruct the midwives in those aspects of nursing that they did not learn in their midwifery training.[59] The Commission agreed, recommending that the Governors of the Rotunda

> at the first opportunity appoint as superintendent of nurses a lady trained in general nursing, so that women coming to the Rotunda for training as mid-wives might be instructed in a part of their business which they do not necessarily learn in their midwifery course.[60]

At the Coombe Hospital, pupil nurses undertook a six-month training period, after which time they received a 'diploma or certificate' of training as a midwife, and the hospital had both internal and external pupil nurses. Internal pupils lived in the hospital and paid a fee of eighteen guineas, eight of which went to the Master as a fee for instruction. External pupils were in the majority and paid a fee of six guineas to the Master. The Commission expressed disappointment that external pupil nurses were not afforded the same opportunity for clinical instruc-tion as the internal pupils. There was no lady superintendent and the pupils were under the charge of the Matron.

Recommendations of the Dublin Hospitals Commission

In its report, the Dublin Hospitals Commission observed that Dublin possessed a large number of hospitals when compared with other cities such as Edinburgh. It reasoned that this could be accounted for in the fact that many hospitals owed their origin to 'the instinct of benevolence' in the previous century and in the fact that Dublin possessed a larger proportion of poor than comparable cities. In addi-tion, many of the Dublin hospitals were founded in the interest of the advancement of medical science, while the Catholic hospitals were founded partly through religious zeal and partly to offer Roman Catholic medical men the means of acquiring an education and a professional reputation. The Commission concluded that the Parliamentary grants to the Dublin hospitals should be contin-ued, on the principle that the funding of hospitals ought to be derived in part from the general taxation of the country, and on the grounds that 'their with-drawal would be attended with most disastrous consequences'. However, the Commission felt obliged to justify the continuance of the Parliamentary grants and attached a precondition upon the hospitals concerned:

> But while we believe that the continuance of the State aid can be justified upon the ground upon which we rely, we concede at once that, before it is sanctioned, the State must be fully satisfied that the reforms which such aid is intended to promote, are likely to be accomplished.[61]

The Commission recommended that the grant be paid to a central fund, which would be administered by Trustees and a Central Board for distribution. This Board would be representative of all parties interested in hospital management, including the Dublin Hospital Sunday Fund, the Dublin Corporation, the three

Dublin medical schools, and the heads of the three main churches in Dublin. The Parliamentary grant would be combined with the Dublin Corporation grant and the funds of the DHSF, in order to generate a single central fund.[62] To be eligible for a share of the proposed fund, each hospital should meet a number of specific conditions relating to its size, function and staffing. The Commission set down six conditions that should be observed by hospitals applying for a share of the fund. A hospital should contain not less than one hundred beds in daily occupation, be open for clinical instruction, have not less than fifty paying students on its books, be open to all creeds without any distinction, and employ staff 'without distinction of creed or of place of education'. The sixth and final condition concerned the nursing arrangements:

> The hospital shall employ as nurses only such persons as have gone through a duly recognized probationary system.[63]

The Commission went on to recommend that the amount of monies to be allocated to any one hospital should be decided upon by a number of considerations that included the number of beds occupied, the 'general efficiency' of the institution, the number of medical students receiving instruction, and the number of 'trained and probationary' nurses.

At a meeting on 10 August 1887, the Council of the DHSF considered the report of the Dublin Hospitals Commission and the proposal for a Dublin Hospital Board Bill, which resulted from the publication of the Commission's report and which provided for the establishment of a Dublin Hospital Board to undertake the distribution of the Parliamentary grants.[64] Since the bill was effectively proposing the assimilation of the funds of the DHSF into a central fund, it implied the de facto removal of the DHSF's independence in the distribution of its grants. The Council of the DHSF resolved that the 'subscribers of the Fund would not consent to entrust the management of the Fund to the proposed Board', advising the promoters of the bill that they 'must not reckon upon the Hospital Sunday Fund forming any part of the proposed revenue of the Board'.[65] As it transpired, the Dublin Hospital Board Bill did not become law and the DHSF continued to function as an independently constituted fundraising movement.[66]

Influence of the Dublin Hospitals Commission

Like the DHSF's Report of the Committee on Nursing of 1879, the report of the Dublin Hospitals Commission highlighted deficiencies in the nursing arrangements at certain Dublin hospitals. However, the Commission's report did not paint such an altogether negative picture as that presented in the report of the DHSF. The Commission praised those hospitals that had reformed their nursing arrangements and it endorsed the recommendations contained in the DHSF report, re-stating the specific recommendation that sick nursing should be carried out by properly trained nurses. Like the DHSF, the Dublin Hospitals Commission also linked eligibility for the awarding of its grants to the extent of hospitals' compliance with its recommendations.

Given the threat of having funds withheld, hospitals that had not introduced reforms at the time when the Commission issued its report now felt obliged to take steps to reform their nursing arrangements. As the only wholly publicly funded institution and the institution in receipt of the largest of the Parliamentary grants awarded to the Dublin hospitals, the Dublin House of Industry Hospitals was quickest to respond to the recommendations of the Commission. In 1888, the Board of Governors appointed Jane Eleanor Hughes and Annie Maria McDonnell as superintendents of nurses and instituted probationership training shortly thereafter. While it is probable that the Catholic Archbishop of Dublin requested the congregations of the Sisters of Mercy and the Irish Sisters of Charity to institute nurse training for Catholic lay nurses at their hospitals, the report of the Commission most likely influenced the decision by the Catholic hospitals to institute nurse training schemes after 1887.[67] In 1891, the Sisters of Mercy established training schools for lay probationers at both the Charitable Infirmary and the Mater Misericordiae Hospital. While St Vincent's Hospital was not the subject of the Commission's inquiries, the Irish Sisters of Charity founded a school of nursing for lay probationers at St Vincent's in 1892.

The Board of Superintendence of Dublin Hospitals

Established on a recommendation of the South Commission in 1856, the Board of Superintendence of Dublin Hospitals was a statutory body with the power to inspect all of the Dublin hospitals in receipt of the Dublin Corporation grant and the Parliamentary grant. The Board of Superintendence had a membership of twelve that included representatives of the boards of management of the hospitals being inspected and it had extensive powers of inquiry. Commencing in 1858, the Board of Superintendence published an annual report, which included commentary on the general state and organization of the Dublin hospitals.[68] Its annual report was the chief means through which it expressed its monitoring function, and the Board was influential in shaping hospital management policy in the second half of the nineteenth century. It was normal practice to have the annual report of the Board of Superintendence laid before the board of management of each Dublin hospital for its consideration. While the annual reports were not in and of themselves instrumental in effecting nursing reform, the Board's inspection function served as a watchdog of standards in hospital management, including hospital sanitation and nursing arrangements.

The influence of the Board of Superintendence was in part a function of its composition, since the representatives of the various Dublin hospitals that sat on the Board could act to ensure that, through the inspection process, improvements could be effected in their respective institutions. Through its annual inspections, the Board succeeded in procuring a number of important reforms in hospital management, including the enforcement of a proper hospital registry, the classification of patients, improvements in accounting and economy, and improvements in dietary arrangements and hospital sanitation. The Board of Superintendence made frequent references to the nursing arrangements in the Dublin hospitals, pointing to deficiencies where these were seen to exist and offering commendations where these were merited. In its Annual Report of 1890, the Board remarked on the nursing arrangements at the Meath Hospital:

> the employment of a superior class of nurses continues to give satisfaction. They appear to be earnest, intelligent and painstaking. [69]

Conclusions

The voluntary hospital was a constitutionally independent institution that, in principle, was largely free to operate its policies in the way that its board of management saw fit. However, in practice, its independence was somewhat nominal, since the voluntary hospital was answerable to the constituency that provided and controlled its funds. Both the Catholic and Protestant voluntary hospitals received a large proportion of their funding from public funds, including the annual Parliamentary and Corporation grants, and from public subscriptions donated through charitable fundraising. The DHSF was the most important source of charitable funds for the Protestant hospitals. In consequence of their control of funding, bodies like Parliament, the Dublin Corporation and the DHSF were in a position to set down a great part of the voluntary hospitals' management policy, including nursing policy.

While both Catholic and Protestant hospitals were answerable to the same constituency of statutory public bodies, the Catholic hospitals were owned and managed by the religious congregations that had founded them and they were also under the influence of the Catholic hierarchy.[70] These institutions maintained a stance of relative independence, both in their dealings with the State and in their general disposition towards the wider developments in hospital management in the period, and this stance of independence would remain a feature of their management style into the twentieth century.[71] Nevertheless, like their Protestant counterparts that depended on public subscriptions, the Catholic hospitals could not be wholly independent.

The quasi-official inquiry by the DHSF Committee on Nursing and the official inquiry of the Dublin Hospitals Commission highlighted deficiencies in the nursing arrangements in the Dublin hospitals in the last quarter of the nineteenth century. While the hospitals associated with the DHSF responded in different ways to the recommendations of the Committee on Nursing, within a relatively short period of time, the majority had reformed their nursing arrangements along the lines recommended.[72] The Dublin Hospitals Commission endorsed the recommendations of the DHSF Committee on Nursing by praising those hospitals that had reformed their nursing arrangements and it called on all hospitals to employ only properly trained nurses. The influence of the Commission was in the fact that it brought those hospitals not operating modern nursing arrangements into line with the Protestant voluntary hospitals that had instituted reforms. In particular, it obliged the Catholic hospitals to introduce systematic training for lay nurses and to employ only properly trained nurses.

In highlighting deficiencies in the nursing arrangements, the DHSF Committee on Nursing report of 1879 provided the voluntary hospitals with a model for nursing and sanitary reform.[73] That model was the system of 'lady nursing' that was built around the Nightingale secular-professional model of pro-bationership training. The model helped to transform nursing from being a form of domestic service to being a respected female occupation and it became the basis for all future developments in nursing.[74] As the Dublin hospitals set about reforming their nursing arrangements in line with the recommendations of the Committee on Nursing and the Dublin Hospitals Commission, they were aware of the success of the Nightingale project of reform in the English voluntary hospitals. The project of nursing reform would became an important part of the business of Dublin's voluntary hospitals in the last two decades of the nineteenth century, when they would experience a transition from an old to a new system of hospital nursing.

3 Hospitals in transition

Two case studies of nursing reform

In the wake of the publication of the influential reports on the nursing arrangements in the Dublin hospitals by the Dublin Hospital Sunday Fund in 1879 and the Dublin Hospitals Commission in 1887, nursing reform became an imperative for the Dublin hospitals. Responding to the calls for the employment of a 'better class' of nurse, properly trained in sick nursing, the members of the boards of management of the voluntary hospitals in Dublin quickly set about the task of putting in place new nursing arrangements. In their task, they were supported by medical men and by a cadre of new nursing managers, the lady superintendents, who were introduced as a prelude to the reforms.

The dual projects of nursing and sanitary reform were major undertakings for Dublin's voluntary hospitals during the 1880s, taking up a considerable amount of the time and energies of their boards of management. Reformers in Dublin took the Nightingale model of nursing reform as their model of reform. The model had its origins in the so-called 'Nightingale experiment', which began at St Thomas's Hospital in the 1860s and which was quickly extended to the other principal voluntary hospitals in London.[1] Two key elements of the Nightingale model of reform were the replacement of the untrained nurse of the servant class with a 'lady nurse' of the middle class, and the introduction of probationership-training schemes. Systematic nurse training was thus an integral part of the project of reform.

What were the experiences of the Dublin hospitals as they set about reforming their nursing arrangements and what were the particular ways in which individual hospitals underwent the transition from the old to the new system? The cases of the two Dublin hospitals, the City of Dublin Hospital and the Dublin House of Industry Hospitals, are used to illustrate the experience of transition for hospitals. The case studies highlight the roles played by the new lady superintendents and illustrate the conflicts and tensions that attended the process of reform.

The City of Dublin Hospital and the City of Dublin Nursing Institution

Four medical men of the Royal College of Surgeons in Ireland founded the City of Dublin Hospital as a clinical teaching hospital in 1832. During the nineteenth century, the hospital developed a reputation as a clinical school for operative surgery and, by the late nineteenth century, was one of the foremost institutions for medical education in Dublin.[2] The hospital was located at Baggot Street, just south of the Grand Canal in a prosperous part of south Dublin, and it was a participating hospital of the DHSF movement.

Like the other Dublin voluntary hospitals in the first half of the nineteenth century, the City of Dublin Hospital relied upon a small and largely untrained nursing workforce to provide the nursing service in its wards. Up until the late 1870s, the hospital continued to employ a matron who was not a trained nurse. At that time, its nurses were described as being 'of the ancient type' and the nursing system was characterized as being the 'old inefficient one'.[3] In common with the other Dublin hospitals in receipt of a grant from the DHSF, the nursing arrangements at the City of Dublin were the subject of the Fund's Committee on Nursing report of 1879. In its report, the Committee identified deficiencies in the system of nursing at the hospital; the supervision of nurses was under the control of a person untrained in the management of the sick and the hospital employed untrained nurses. There were no arrangements for the systematic training of nurses and there were deficiencies in nurses' accommodation, wages and recreation. In common with most other hospitals at that time, 'the only qualification absolutely required for nurses previous to appointment [at the City of Dublin Hospital was] ... good character and ability to read and write'.[4]

In their annual report for the year 1878, the Board of Directors of the hospital had described the nursing arrangements at the hospital as being 'very good: the Hospital having nine Trained Nurses, two Assistants, and five Wardmaids'.[5] However, the Board pointed to a lack of accommodation for nurses and indicated their intention to obtain more space when funds became available. The report of the DHSF Committee on Nursing was laid before the Board at its meeting of 11 March 1879. In responding to the report, the Board resolved to correct the deficiencies in the hospital's nursing arrangements and they moved quickly to improve matters, establishing an internal committee to inquire into the nursing arrangements.[6] This committee reported back to the Board of Directors on 4 April, proposing that one of the hospital wards be given over to the nurses as sleeping accommodation. The Board accepted the proposal and converted Dr Storey's Female Eye Ward to accommodate the nurses. The Board was now in a position to respond to the DHSF, stating:

> so far as possible they have carried out the suggestions made by ... [the Committee on Nursing] and they have now provided increased accommodation for nurses by turning one of the wards into a bedroom for the nurses.[7]

In their annual report for the year 1879, the Board of Directors was in a position to describe the nursing arrangements as being 'excellent'; nine trained nurses were employed and additional sleeping accommodation was provided for them on the recommendation of the DHSF.[8] In 1882, two additional trained nurses were appointed.

In May 1883, the Dublin Nurses' Training Institution at Holles Street made a proposal to the Board of Directors of the City of Dublin Hospital to enter into an arrangement wherein the nurses of the Institution would receive practical training in the wards of the hospital. The Board agreed that it would be 'an advantage to the hospital to … allow the Nurses' Institute (sic) the privilege of training probationers in this hospital'.[9] The proposal would entail the appointment of a lady superintendent of nursing, her salary to be paid by the Institution and her accommodation to be provided by the hospital, and six probationers would be trained annually under the lady superintendent. In September 1883, the Board recommended the appointment of a lady superintendent along with two head nurses at a salary of £20 each per annum. However, in a counter proposal, William deCourcy Wheeler, a surgeon at the hospital, proposed:

> [the establishment of] a Nursing Institution in connection with the City of Dublin Hospital … to improve the nursing department of the Hospital, to train suitable persons as nurses for the Hospital [and] to train suitable persons to attend as Medical, Surgical or Fever nurses in private families.[10]

Mr deCourcy Wheeler also proposed the appointment of a lady superintendent who would have control over the entire nursing staff of the hospital. The hospital would provide 'every facility for training' and probationers would 'live in the vicinity of the hospital under the surveillance of the lady superintendent'. Though financially independent, the proposed institution would be 'especially associated' with the hospital. In its deliberations on the proposal, the Board of Directors resolved that it would be important to secure the establishment of the proposed training institution, and it accepted Mr deCourcy Wheeler's proposal under the condition that it be brought into existence by 1 January 1884. Further consideration of the proposal from the Dublin Nurses' Training Institution at Holles Street was deferred.

Wishing to 'raise the nursing of the Hospital to the highest attainable efficiency', the Board of Directors announced in its annual report for 1883 the establishment of the City of Dublin Nursing Institution.[11] The *Rules for the Regulation of the Training Institution* were drawn up and presented to the Board at its meeting in November 1883, and the City of Dublin Nursing Institution 'for training women as nurses for the sick in hospitals and in private families' was formally constituted.[12] In December, Miss Susan Beresford, formerly the Lady Superintendent at Sir Patrick Dun's Hospital, was approved for appointment as Lady Superintendent and the Secretary of the Board notified the Dublin Hospital Sunday Fund of the appointment. The Lady Superintendent was responsible for the entire nursing department of the hospital and for the new City of Dublin Nursing Institution. The Matron of the hospital, Mrs Finlay, who held the titles of Lady Superintendent and Matron, would now hold only the title of Matron.

The City of Dublin Nursing Institution, under the management of a Board of Directors drawn from the City of Dublin Hospital, was established at premises

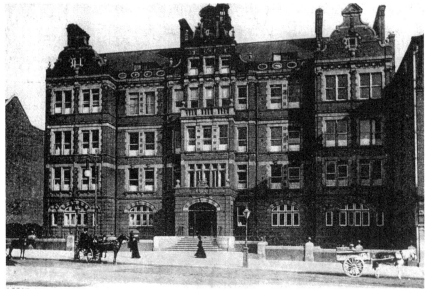

Figure 3.1 City of Dublin Hospital, Baggot Street, *c.*1900. Courtesy of the Irish Historical
Picture Company

opposite the Hospital at 27 Upper Baggot Street. The *Regulations of the City of
Dublin Nursing Institution Limited* were placed before the Board of the Hospital on 8
February 1884.[13] The regulations contained details of the conditions of training
for probationers of the Institution, including the entry requirements:

> They must be over eighteen years and under forty years of age at the date of
> application. They must be able to read and write well, and bring testimonials
> of good character.[14]

Applicants would be placed on a three-month probationary period and would
receive a salary of £10 for the first year, £15 per annum for three years, and £20
per annum if engaged for a second period of three years. A certificate would be
granted on the completion of each term of three years and 'special diplomas …
awarded when deserved'. The regulations advised intending applicants that probationers 'must attend and do duty as Nurses in the City of Dublin Hospital or
elsewhere, as they may be directed [and] must obey such directions and instructions as may be given them during their training'. Nurses and probationers would
be provided with a home, boarding, and washing. The regulations prohibited the
receiving of gratuities from patients and the use of wine or spirits, and probationers were 'subject to instant dismissal for disobedience of orders, culpable neglect,
or other misconduct'. Prospective candidates were cautioned that 'any misbehav-
iour or want of attention on the part of a nurse [would] be at once reported to the
Lady Superintendent or to the Secretary'.

New arrangements for nursing

The inauguration of the City of Dublin Nursing Institution as a training school was somewhat inauspicious. The newly appointed Lady Superintendent Miss Beresford advised the Board of Directors that she had difficulty accepting the *Rules and Regulations of the City of Dublin Nursing Institution* and she offered her resignation to the Board on the grounds that she could not act under the rules. Miss Beresford's particular difficulty was in the fact that the rules gave the Directors of the Institution and not herself the power to dismiss nurses and she advised the Board:

> I must have the power to engage and dismiss nurses otherwise how could I possibly be responsible for the Nursing.[15]

Miss Beresford insisted that 'no Lady who has had any experience of the great difficulties of a training school would work under such rules'. Her resignation was accepted, and at a special meeting of the Board on 15 February 1884, the names of three other persons, Miss Bewley of Doncaster General Infirmary, Miss Hamilton of the London Hospital, and Miss Haipin of the Pendlebury Hospital, Manchester, were put forward for consideration as suitable candidates for the post of Lady Superintendent.[16]

Miss Susanne Helena Bewley was selected and duly appointed as Lady Superintendent on 22 February 1884 under new conditions of employment, which set out her duties at both the City of Dublin Hospital and the City of Dublin Nursing Institution. At the hospital, she would 'superintend and have the immediate control of the Nurses, Assistant Nurses, Probationers and Ward Maids, in all matters relating to their Hospital duties'.[17] She should also take charge of and be responsible for the training of all probationers engaged in the hospital, carefully attending to their instruction and giving them 'all proper opportunities of learning their duties as Nurses'. At the City of Dublin Nursing Institution, she should 'take charge and be responsible for the transaction of the business of the Institution in reference to the hiring out of nurses and the training of Probationers'. Miss Bewley was also given the authority to suspend any nurse, assistant nurse, probationer or wardmaid in the service of the hospital or Nursing Institution for 'misconduct or negligence, insubordination, or disobedience to her orders'.

Miss Bewley took up her duties in February 1884 and by March she had dismissed as 'unsuitable for the post' nurse Bessie Fleming in Drummond Wing. In April, in 'compliance with the wishes of Drs Benson and Duffy', she presided over two further dismissals, those of a night nurse and the nurse in charge of the fever ward, and she instituted improvements in the sanitation of the wards of the hospital. In April, Miss Bewley presented a detailed report on the hospital's nursing arrangements to the Board of Directors.[18] In her report, she gave details of further dismissals, including those of the nurse on the male surgical ward for 'negligence and impertinence to one of the members of the Surgical staff' and the nurse in the female surgical and gynaecological wards, 'on account of gross impropriety of conduct'. She recommended that Nurse Kellett, having spent twenty-two years in the service of the hospital, be permitted to retire with a retiring allowance in recognition of the long and faithful discharge of her duties. In her report, Miss Bewley noted that probationers of the City of Dublin Nursing Institution were now available for nursing duties at the hospital. She proposed that the nursing could be effectually carried out by appointing a properly trained and qualified nurse to act as Head Nurse and by two staff nurses who would work with the assistance of probationers:

> to ensure the success of this plan, it would be necessary that the 2 staff nurses should be superior women fully trained and qualified capable also of instructing Probationers, winning their respect and obedience.[19]

In order to obtain such women, she recommended that the salary of £13 per annum be increased to at least £25. Night nurses should also receive an improved salary.

Miss Bewley found as objectionable the practice of the night nurse on the male division having to open the hall door at night, on the grounds that the nurse was forced to leave cases of extreme urgency and even to leave the dying unattended. Two trained nurses assisted by probationers could do the night nursing more efficiently, she suggested, and the 'very responsible position' of night nurse should be filled by women 'who could be depended upon and necessarily of a better class than those now employed in the Hospital, upon whom I could not place any reliance'. Concluding her report to the Board, Miss Bewley declared:

> If this arrangement is approved … I will undertake with the assistance given by the Probationers, that the nursing of the Hospital will be performed in a thoroughly satisfactory manner and by 6 Hospital Nurses instead of 9 … Notwithstanding the increase in the individual wages it will be more economical for the Hospital, I also believe that the patients will be better attended to, the directions of the staff more strictly and efficiently carried out, the wards better kept and the general tone of the Hospital in every way improved.[20]

The Board of Directors adopted Miss Bewley's report on the nursing arrangements, including her proposals for change. The reforms that were instituted had a marked effect in the hospital wards and, in its annual report for the year 1884, the Board of Directors declared:

> The new system of nursing … was inaugurated this year. A marked improvement in the cleanliness and comfort of the wards, and, consequently, of the patients, has taken place; and the bright faces and neat dresses of the probationers are cheering to the poor sick recipients of this service.[21]

The reforms also involved the introduction of a new set of rules for the hospital Matron, which made her responsible for the entire household management and domestic arrangements and superintending all the servants, but not including the nurses, assistant nurses, probationers and wardmaids, who would thereafter be the responsibility of the Lady Superintendent.[22]

Although brief, Helena Bewley's tenure as Lady Superintendent was productive in effecting improvements in the nursing arrangements and the Board of Directors accepted with regret her resignation in December 1884. Miss Susan Beresford, who had previously declined to take up the position of Lady Superintendent, was appointed as her successor in early 1885. In the same year, having 'served the hospital faithfully for twenty-two years', the Matron Mrs Finlay retired and was succeeded as Matron by Mrs Fry.[23]

The first cohort of probationers from the City of Dublin Nursing Institution completed their training in 1886 and nurses Fitzgerald and Haughton were among the first probationers of the Institution to be appointed as staff nurses at the hospital.[24] The Board of Directors remarked that the 'the skilled hands of the Staff Nurses, and the cheerful services of the probationers' went far to aid the work of the physicians and surgeons.[25] In 1887, Miss Beresford resigned her position as Lady Superintendent of the City of Dublin Nursing Institution and assumed the position of Lady Superintendent for the City of Dublin Hospital alone. During her tenure, Miss Beresford presided over the consolidation of the new nursing arrangements, which had given 'entire satisfaction'.[26] By the early 1890s, a total of thirty-six probationers and sixty-three qualified nurses were working in the service of the hospital and in private cases.[27] Miss Beresford resigned as Lady Superintendent in 1896 and was replaced by Miss Helen Shuter, who had trained at St Thomas's and St Bartholomew's hospitals in London.

In the 1890s, the City of Dublin Nursing Institution had become so important a part of the City of Dublin Hospital that it was considered to be 'materially a portion of its latter-day history'.[28] During this period Mrs J. Kildare Treacy, one of the first students to train at the City of Dublin Hospital, was Lady Manager of the Institution. In 1893, following a recommendation from the Visiting Committee of the DHSF, the hospital undertook major redevelopments that included new nurses' accommodation.[29] When the Visiting Committee returned in 1894, it reported that 'nothing better could be desired … the [nurses' home is the] picture of comfort'.[30]

When a contingent of five nurses from the City of Dublin Nursing Institution joined the Army Nursing Service Reserve in 1899 to travel to the Boer War in South Africa, a newspaper report carried the following accolade:

> In addition to complying with regulations, which define an extremely high standard of professional training and experience, these nurses have fully satisfied the severest tests … Four continuous years combined hospital training and nursing service, a complete systematic course of instruction, hospital work in medical, surgical and fever wards, two examinations and experience in positions of trust and responsibility, with exemplary conduct and character, and proved ability to endure hard work and to undertake responsibility, constitute the conditions upon which they have been chosen.[31]

In October 1899, the hospital decided to terminate its arrangement with the City of Dublin Nursing Institution and to establish its own nurse training school. The new training school was duly established in February 1900 and a new nurses' home was opened in 1902, providing accommodation for thirty-five nurses and probationers. The Visiting Committee of the DHSF reported that the new home was 'lit all over with electric light, and all the arrangements in it are first rate'.[32] By 1910, the total number of probationers available for duty in the service of the hospital was twenty-nine.[33]

The Dublin House of Industry Hospitals

The Dublin House of Industry was opened in 1773 on the north bank of the river Liffey at North Brunswick Street as the workhouse of the Corporation for the Relief of the Poor in Dublin.[34] Opened as a pauper institution, the Dublin House of Industry was effectively the poor house for the greater part of Dublin and, like the workhouses of the nineteenth century, it functioned as an institution for medical relief; as early as 1774, two wards were opened for the accommodation of medical and surgical patients.[35] The institution was initially supported by charitable contributions and by the award of an annual Parliamentary grant. By the time of the publication of the Dublin Hospitals Commission in 1887, the institution was in receipt of the largest of the Parliamentary grants awarded to the Dublin hospitals.[36] The institution was not a participant hospital in the Dublin Hospital Sunday Fund movement.

In the early nineteenth century, there developed a number of hospitals directly associated with the Dublin House of Industry at or near to the North Brunswick Street site. These included the Hardwicke Fever Hospital (1803), the Bedford Asylum for Children (1806), the Richmond Surgical Hospital and the Talbot Dispensary (1811), the Whitworth Medical Hospital (1817), and the Richmond Lunatic Asylum at Grangegorman (1814).[37] With the enactment of the Poor Relief (Ireland) Act in 1838, much of the original building became the North Dublin Union Workhouse and the hospitals came under the control of the Poor Law Commissioners. However, following a recommendation of the South Commission in 1856, the Commissioners of Public Works assumed control over the hospitals, a Board of Governors was appointed by the Lord Lieutenant and the constituent hospitals were separated from the poor law system.[38]

The Dublin House of Industry became a prominent institution for medical relief for the sick poor of Dublin and it became an important clinical hospital of the Dublin School, where students received lectures 'upon all branches of medical and surgical science'.[39] In 1854, the House of Commons Select Committee on Dublin Hospitals reported that the Dublin House of Industry, containing a fever hospital and a hospital for chronic medical disease, was considered to be the best institution by far in Dublin suited for the purpose of clinical instruction.[40]

The Dublin House of Industry was essentially 'one institution, under three roofs'.[41] By the 1870s, the Richmond, Hardwicke and Whitworth hospitals had a combined total of 312 beds, providing for the treatment of surgical, medical and fever cases.[42] The constituent hospitals provided medical relief for the population of over one hundred thousand on the north side of the city that included the families of soldiers in the Royal Barracks, traders in the Smithfield markets, poor arriving on the train from the west of Ireland, and emigrants and crews of ships at the quays to the east.[43] With its role as a clinical hospital of the Dublin School and with its prominent role in medical relief, the Dublin House of Industry pursued the projects of nursing and sanitary reform. However, unlike its counterpart at Baggot Street, this institution's transition from the old to the new system of hospital nursing was rather protracted and tortuous.

Early attempts at reform

In the decade immediately prior to the widespread movement for nursing reform in Dublin, the nursing care at the Dublin House of Industry Hospitals was carried out by nurses who were untrained, mostly illiterate, and usually recruited from the ranks of the wardmaids. The Matron was Mrs Annie Byrne. Appointed in 1870 and having served for seven years as the Matron of Mountjoy Prison, Mrs Byrne had come to the Dublin House of Industry with the 'experience of maintaining discipline, cleanliness and tidiness'.[44] She lived with her children at the hospital and, in common with her counterparts in most of the Dublin hospitals in the period, she was not herself a trained nurse. She was, however, described as 'a most excellent officer … able and zealous'.[45]

Much of Mrs Byrne's time was taken with applying sanctions for breaches of discipline by the nurses in her charge and with bringing her reports of these breaches to the attention of the Board of Governors. The most common form of sanction for neglect of duty was a fine and a reprimand and, for serious breaches of discipline, dismissal. In August 1871, the Governors considered Mrs Byrne's report, which noted that a Nurse Turner's inefficiency was 'becoming everyday more embarrassing to her'.[46] Along with nurses Caldwell and Rutledge, Turner was implicated in the pilfering of hospital stock. The Governors ordered that Turner be replaced and that reprimands and a fine of two shillings each be issued to Nurse Caldwell and to four wardmaids for 'being in bed at 10 minutes to 7 o'clock … when they should have been on duty from 6 o'clock'. On visiting the Hardwicke Hospital at 10.30 in the evening of 15 March 1878, Mrs Byrne found Nurse McEvoy of 4 Division Hardwicke and the night nurse Sarah Bannister under the influence of drink. Both were suspended and they later resigned. In the following year, a group of nurses was fined for 'disobedience in going into each others closets for the purpose of gossiping'.

The practice of promoting wardmaids to the position of nurse was also part of the duties of the Matron. In September 1871, Mrs Byrne promoted wardmaid Charlotte Brophy to the position of night nurse in the Richmond Hospital and replaced her with Catherine Kenna. Kenna did not fare well in her new position as wardmaid, and was fined two shillings for being in bed at 2 o'clock in the afternoon, for failing to help with the work, and for being 'very indolent'. While it was possible to be promoted from wardmaid to nurse, the reverse was also possible and it appears that, under Mrs Byrne, the positions were interchangeable. For example, in October 1880, nurse Darby was demoted to the position of ward-maid for being under the influence of drink.

An initiative to improve the nursing arrangements began in May 1881, when the physicians and surgeons, through a letter to their Honorary Secretary Dr Gordon, advised the Board of Governors:

> Some very decided change is required in the nursing of patients in the Richmond Hospital, and they recommend that a fully qualified Head Nurse shall be immediately appointed.[47]

In response, the Board resolved that in future only trained nurses should be appointed to vacancies in the nursing department. When the Board advertised for trained nurses, of the six candidates who applied, only one, Martha Massey, was a trained nurse. Massey did not attend for interview and instead Eliza Jones, not herself a trained nurse, was appointed. Mary Molloy, also untrained as a nurse, was engaged as night nurse at the Whitworth, but was discharged less than a month later for being asleep in bed while on duty. When the Governors succeeded in recruiting a trained and certified nurse for the Whitworth Hospital in 1884, the appointment was short-lived; Mary Burns, the nurse appointed, died of Typhus Fever in January 1885.

In 1885, when the Dublin Hospitals Commission visited the Hospital, the surgeons continued to press for changes to the nursing arrangements and the Board of Governors responded with a novel way of improving the situation.[48] Perhaps mindful of the risk of losing the Parliamentary grant, the Governors proposed a way of ensuring that its nurses could be deemed to be 'qualified'. On the basis of a complaint received from Mr Stokes about the nursing at the Richmond Hospital, one Board member Mr Charles E. Martin tabled a motion that would recognize the nurses as trained nurses:

> It having been conveyed to the Board by Mr Stokes some of the Nurses in the Richmond Hospital are untrained and inefficient – the Board now beg to call attention of the surgical staff to the matter … The Board consider that any Nurse who has had the advantage of serving under the distinguished Surgeons and efficient staff of this Hospital, should, after a sufficient lapse of time, be thereby highly qualified and efficient in every aspect.[49]

Along with attempting to confer responsibility for the training of nurses onto the surgeons, it appears that Mr Martin was also attempting to pre-empt the Dublin Hospitals Commission in relation to questions that might arise concerning the nursing arrangements, and he was seeking to present the institution in the best possible light for the Commission.

'A better state of things'

With the publication of the Report of the Dublin Hospitals Commission in 1887 and the Commission's finding that the nursing arrangements at the Dublin House of Industry Hospitals were not satisfactory, the need to reform was clear. The Board of Governors moved quickly and appointed a Special Committee of Inspection 'to investigate the general management of the House of Industry Hospitals and to suggest improvements if necessary'. Comprising members of the Board and medical staff, the Special Committee presented its report to the Board with recommendations that it considered would 'help to a better state of things'.[50]

Dated 22 February 1888, much of the report was concerned with household arrangements, such as the condition of the wards, bathrooms and kitchens. In the Richmond Hospital, the bathroom was reported as being 'very dirty ... [and] No. 1 ward [was] dirty and untidy'. The report described the conditions in No. 1 ward:

> The floor had not been waxed for some time. The patients' tables were unclean; broken bread, in one case a piece of cold breakfast, medicine bottles, bits of newspapers, &c., lay in confusion upon them. The water-closet opens directly upon the ward. It was in a shocking state. Urine lay all over the floor, and the W. C. contained a quantity of filth. A few chamber pots, some with urine, lay on the floor. The stench was very bad.[51]

The wards on the second floor were found to be cleaner and tidier, while the third floor was 'clean, but might be cleaner'. The report on the conditions of the wards in the Whitworth and Hardwicke Hospitals also painted a picture of disarray and uncleanness:

> There is no fixed bath in the Whitworth ... The water-closets are better than in the Richmond, but they need repairs ... The water-closet outside the Hardwicke is in a filthy condition ... The night nurse's sleeping room is uncurtained and is open to outside inspection. There is but one bath in the Hardwicke and it is inefficient.[52]

The Special Committee wrote that despite concerns of the physicians and surgeons some years previously concerning the appointment of nurses, 'incompetent persons have been appointed without any reference to them whatever'. In its report, the Special Committee indicated where it believed the solution to the problems lay, making a deliberate reference to the nursing arrangements:

> It is clear that the supervision of the nurses is not as complete as is necessary, and that the nursing staff is altogether insufficient. Each nurse is practically independent, with the exception of such intermittent supervision as the matron is able to give. This was made evident by the state of the wards, and the dirty hands and faces of some of the patients, who, not being able to leave their beds, did not have any particular attention paid to their cleanliness.[53]

The Special Committee went on to make very specific recommendations on the nursing arrangements:

> We are of the opinion that a highly qualified nurse should be appointed to both the Richmond and the Whitworth Hospitals, each with charge of the nursing staff, and the general orderliness and discipline of her hospital. The number of nurses should be increased, either by trained nurses, or by probationers.[54]

The Special Committee advised that, pending completion of some arrangement of the sort proposed, no nurse should be appointed without first having the approval of the physicians and surgeons. It recommended improvements in sanitation, heating, lighting and cooking and, while it acknowledged that it did not expect all of the changes to be made at once, the Special Committee expressed its 'strong opinion ... that the present staff is one which needs re-organization with a view to the better nursing of patients'.

Mrs Byrne interpreted the report of the Special Committee as a criticism of her personally, and she forwarded a lengthy and detailed reply to the Board of Governors entitled 'Matron's Explanation'.[55] In her reply, she addressed each finding in the report. She gave the reasons why, in her view, the Committee members found what they did, and she sought to explain and/or to challenge the findings of the report. Refuting the finding that the supervision of nurses was incomplete, she declared:

> The nurses are not independent of me, they are under my control as well as the wardmaids and other servants, and so intimate am I with the business character of each one that I know which, if any is an eye-servant, and consequently know when and where to make an unexpected visit. I must say that in justice to them that as a rule I find them attentive to their duties and discharging them to the best of their ability ...[56]

Mrs Byrne called on the Board to 'acquit me of all the "dirt" and "filth" attributed to my management in the Report'. She also felt obliged to include a character reference given some years previously by Captain Barlow, Director of Government Prisons and her former employer at Mountjoy, who reported that Mrs Byrne was 'in *every* respect a most *satisfactory* officer'.[57] The Board of Governors replied sympathetically to Mrs Byrne, expressing regret that she was 'under misapprehension as regards the meaning of the report' and, by way of explanation, advised her:

> [The Governors] do not find in the report evidence that anything personal was intended ... and that the alleged defects in the hospitals, pointed out in the report could not be held to be the result of mismanagement on your part.[58]

Mrs Byrne's protest notwithstanding, the Board of Governors adopted the report of the Special Committee, including all of its recommendations.

New superintendents of nurses

At its meeting of March 1888, the Board of Governors resolved to advertise for two trained and certified superintendents of nurses for the Richmond Surgical and the Whitworth Medical hospitals, at a salary of £60 per annum, with rations, light and fuel. Twenty-seven persons replied to the public advertisement and, in April, Jane Eleanor Hughes and Annie Maria McDonnell were appointed as superintendents of nurses at the Whitworth Hospital and Richmond Hospital respectively. The Board of Governors prepared accommodation for the new superintendents, drafted a code of rules for the management of the hospitals, and the Board members duly received Miss Hughes and Miss McDonnell on 11 July 1888. Their duties included being responsible for supervising the nurses and regulating their duties, conduct and dress. While Miss Hughes and Miss McDonnell reported directly to the Board of Governors, Mrs Byrne continued to act as Matron of the Hardwicke Fever Hospital and was placed in charge of the general kitchen and the laundry. In the following year, Mrs Byrne was given charge of mending the linen and thereafter she was effectively Head of Laundry and Head of Kitchen.

Of the two new lady superintendents, Annie McDonnell took the initiative in reforming the nursing and sanitary arrangements. She wasted no time in bringing forward proposals for improving the situation; her report book, which was laid before the Governors in August 1888, contained 'numerous suggestions involving alterations in arrangements for Nurses' and Servants' accommodation, [and] rate of pay for nursing staff'.[59] She proposed the engagement of probationers and 'many other matters, the carrying out of which would entail a very considerable expenditure of money'. In September, she engaged three trained and certified nurses, Cooney, Growney and Clinton, and she directed nurse Julia Callery to act as pupils' servant, but later dismissed her along with Julia Hayden for 'drunkenness and incapacity'. By November, she had a complement of four day nurses and two night nurses, had implemented improvements in the nurses' living arrangements, and selected a new nurse's uniform. She called for the employment of a hall porter during night time, in order to permit the night nurse on the lower division of the Richmond to give her time to her nursing duties. She called for improved wages for the nurses, advising the Governors that the wages paid to nurses were only two-thirds that paid elsewhere to trained nurses. The Governors ordered that Miss McDonnell's plan should be tried for three months in the three hospitals.

With Miss McDonnell's new nursing arrangements in place, the expenditure on nursing had greatly increased and, in March 1889, the Medical Board proposed a solution to the Governors:

> [The Medical Board] cannot see that any reduction in the number of day or night nurses could be made without seriously interfering with the efficiency of the Nursing. In order to lessen expenses, they would suggest, that the system

of Probationership be introduced into these hospitals. Under this system, young women are trained as Nurses in the Hospital, incurring about £10 a year, and after a year's training are bound to remain in the Service of the Hospital for two more years.[60]

The Medical Board went on to outline the benefits of introducing a probationership-training system.

The Medical Board think it would be possible to introduce such a system into these Hospitals, as all the members of the Medical Staff are practising Physicians [and] Surgeons in Dublin. For nurses so trained could be used by them, in their private cases, instead of having to be procured from some other Nursing Institution, to the benefit of the latter.[61]

In May, a Joint Committee of the Visiting Governors and the physicians and surgeons urged the Board of Governors to carry out the proposal to introduce a probationership-training scheme without delay. The Board accepted the proposal and requested the Joint Committee to prepare the necessary rules and conditions in connection with the proposed scheme; the Joint Committee duly prepared the *Rules for Nurses*, which contained the terms under which nurses could be employed.[62] The candidate would serve a one-month trial period, at the end of which the Superintendent of Nurses would decide on her fitness to become a probationer. The training period was one year, after which time the probationer would receive a certificate of training. The Board of Governors accepted the *Rules for Nurses* and, in November, Miss McDonnell reported that two candidates had satisfactorily completed their trial period and were now entered for training as probationer nurses. Miss McDonnell also engaged two new staff nurse sisters for day duty and one new staff nurse sister for night duty, and a third probationer entered training in January 1890.

In May 1890, Mrs Byrne was advised that the Board of Governors had 'finally determined to relieve her from the care of the patients in the Hardwicke Hospital and to ask her careful supervision of all the ordinary duties of Matron, including the Laundry'. Miss Hughes was asked to take charge of the Hardwicke Fever Hospital in addition to her responsibilities at the Whitworth.

The new nursing arrangements were the subject of commentary by the Board of Superintendence of Dublin Hospitals, which noted in its annual report for 1890 that the patients gave satisfactory replies 'when interrogated on the subject of their fare, its cooking, service, and on the attention of the nurses'.[63] The Board of Superintendence reported that 'the nurses are all competent, kind and attentive to the patients; they are under the control of two highly trained Lady Superintendents and a matron of long experience'.

By March 1891, the Dublin House of Industry Hospitals employed a total of forty-six nurses and probationers and its nurses were earning fees from external duties, including private nursing and the provision of a nursing service to prisons and country infirmaries. Reporting on the circumstances of the Dublin House of

Industry Hospitals in 1892, the Board of Superintendence of Dublin Hospitals observed:

> On inspection, we are pleased to find that this Institution continues to be efficiently conducted in all departments, which is in no small degree to be ascribed to the close care and attention given by the Governors to its administration, and also to the improved system of nursing. [64]

Annie McDonnell

During the period when the nursing arrangements were being reformed, there were tensions and conflicts between Mrs Byrne and the two new lady superintendents. In November 1892, Miss McDonnell complained to the Board of Governors that, despite repeated complaints about the matter, the dietary for the nurses 'could not be worse', and she warned:

> Unless some change is made so as to make the nurses necessarily comfortable at their meals, we cannot hope to keep their work up, or to return so good a class of young woman as up to the present we have attained.[65]

The Board took Miss McDonnell's concerns seriously and advised Mrs Byrne that if the dietary for nurses did not improve within six months, she would be requested to resign. Later in January 1894, as part of its 'contemplated changes' in the management of the hospitals, the Board wrote to Mrs Byrne requesting her resignation. Mrs Byrne duly resigned, having been granted a pension for her services 'according

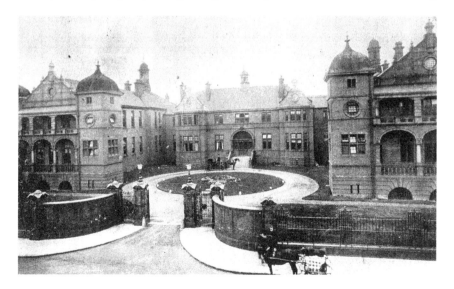

Figure 3.2 New Richmond Hospital, Dublin, *c.*1896. Courtesy of the Irish Historical Picture Company

to the highest scale' and a gratuity of £60. Mrs Byrne had served as Matron for a total of twenty-three years.

In February, a special committee of the Board of Governors met to appoint a successor to Mrs Byrne. The special committee recommended that Miss McDonnell be appointed Lady Superintendent of the three hospitals of the Dublin House of Industry at a salary of £100 per annum. She should have 'supreme control of the nursing staff and female servants [and] she should have the direction of the whole of the nursing and domestic arrangements of the Hospitals, including the Cooking and Laundry Work.'[66] In November, Miss Hughes offered her resignation as Superintendent of Nurses at the Whitworth Medical and Hardwicke Fever hospitals, which the Board accepted with regret.[67] Upon Miss Hughes's resignation, Miss McDonnell was duly appointed Lady Superintendent of the Richmond, Hardwicke and Whitworth Hospitals, where she would go on to provide service for a further twenty years.

A native of Londonderry, Annie McDonnell trained under Margaret Huxley at Sir Patrick Dun's Hospital and, when she first took up her appointment at the Richmond Surgical Hospital, she had the distinction of being 'the first lady nurse trained in Ireland who became a Hospital Superintendent'.[68] Under Annie McDonnell, the Dublin House of Industry became a full participant in the system of probationership training in Dublin, and its nursing arrangements were brought up to the same standard as those obtaining in the other major Dublin voluntary hospitals.[69] Miss McDonnell was a founding member of the first Governing Authority of the Dublin Metropolitan Technical School for Nurses and her probationers attended the school for theoretical instruction. A new nurses' home, described as 'a model of neatness and comfort', was completed in 1896.[70]

Following its annual inspection in 1899, the Board of Superintendence of Dublin Hospitals was once again forthright in its praise for the state of hospital management in the institution:

> It is evident that great energy and earnestness is shown in the general management of this institution … we found the wards clean and in order … The assiduous attention of the Lady Superintendent to the requirements of the patients and the devotion of the nursing staff to their duties leaves nothing to report but what is satisfactory.[71]

During her tenure as Lady Superintendent, Miss McDonnell left the Dublin House of Industry Hospitals for a period of ten months to head up Lord Iveagh's field hospital in the Boer War in South Africa.[72] She and her assistant were the first ladies to enter Pretoria; upon their arrival, Lord Roberts greeted them, exclaiming: 'Well done the Irish!' For her service in the South African War, Annie McDonnell was awarded the South African War Medal and the Royal Red Cross, the highest order of merit a woman could obtain. She was described as 'a woman of exceptional vigour, quick perception, sound principles, physical activity, and healthy constitution'.[73]

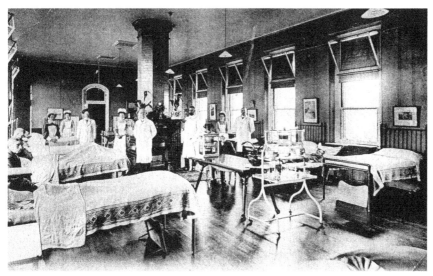

Figure 3.3 'Clean and in order', No. 1 Ward, Richmond Hospital, Dublin, *c*.1900. Courtesy of the Irish Historical Picture Company

When Margaret Huxley retired as a Lady Superintendent, Annie McDonnell was regarded as the 'senior lady nurse in Dublin'.[74] When she herself retired in 1909, she was co-opted as a member of the Board of Superintendence of Dublin Hospitals.[75] Her tenure as Superintendent of Nurses at the Dublin House of Industry Hospitals was summarized in a tribute to her, published at the time of her retirement:

> Miss McDonnell … now retires … after twenty years of arduous work, during which she had to encounter much additional effort and personal responsibility during the transition period in the history of that venerable institution, from a condition in which much of the old world lingered about it outwardly, to its present state of perfection, with all that is up-to-date in modern science secured for it.[76]

The new order

The City of Dublin Hospital and the Dublin House of Industry Hospitals were important institutions for medical relief in Dublin and, by virtue of their roles as clinical hospitals of the Dublin School, were prominent in the movement for nursing and sanitary reform in the last quarter of the nineteenth century. Their respective experiences in reforming their nursing arrangements serve to illustrate the process of transition that they each underwent. In replacing the old system of nursing with the new, the experience of transition for each institution was unique, being moderated by local conditions that were a function of their respective histories. However, there were commonalities in the experience of transition for both institutions, the most notable of which was the almost total replacement of a workforce of largely untrained nurses from the poorer classes with professionally trained nurses recruited from the middle and lower middle classes.

Its prior relationship with the poor law system and its funding arrangements rendered the Dublin House of Industry Hospitals as a wholly public institution. Its status as a public institution contributed to its relatively protracted and tortuous transition to the new order; as a state-funded institution, it could implement major changes in hospital management only with the assent of the Lord Lieutenant. Its more independent counterpart at Baggot Street came under the sphere of influence of the Dublin Hospital Sunday Fund. This fact partly explains why the City of Dublin Hospital had moved with such relative speed to reform its nursing arrangements. The local conditions of each institution were also partly a function of the composition of their respective boards of management. The influence that individual board members wielded in shaping local management policy determined the particular ways in which the reforms were conducted in each hospital; the medical members of the boards of management were among the strongest advocates of nursing reform.

Evidence from the two case studies indicates that the Dublin hospitals experienced a considerable amount of organizational reform in a relatively short period of time. While the pace of reform could vary from one hospital to the next, by the early 1890s, the outcome for all of the Dublin hospitals participating in the reforms was the ending of a system of hospital management that had remained in place since the voluntary hospitals were first opened. In the transition, the new system that replaced the old transformed the care of the hospitalized sick poor, providing them with a greatly improved system of nursing and improved sanitary conditions. In the process, nursing itself was transformed from a low status occupation to one that was considered one of the highest standing for women. The new nursing arrangements that were established in the period laid the foundations for the system of hospital nursing that are recognizable up to the present time.

Lady superintendents

While nursing reform was initiated by Anglican social reformers of the Dublin middle and upper classes that included members of the Anglo-Irish nobility, Anglican clergymen, and Protestant medical men, the cadre of newly appointed nurse managers, the lady superintendents, implemented the reforms. The lady superintendents were well chosen by the hospitals' boards of management and were most capable of effecting radical changes in a relatively short period of time. Official bodies, such as the Dublin Hospitals Commission and the Board of Superintendence of Dublin Hospitals, attested to their capabilities and their achievements were not confined to the introduction of new nursing arrangements, but also included improvements in hospital sanitation and reforms in hospital management more generally. While they were acting at the behest of the men who employed them, the lady superintendents were themselves originators and implementers of much of the management policy and were most capable of acting in ways that they saw fit.

In all of the Dublin hospitals that participated in the reforms, a lady superintendent replaced the untrained matron. The lady superintendents were educated gentlewomen of Anglo-Irish, English or Scottish parentage, and many were the daughters of professionals, including doctors and military officers, or the daughters of country gentlemen. Most received their nurse training in the reformed Anglican voluntary hospitals in London, Manchester and Liverpool. Elinor Lyons, the first Lady Superintendent at the Meath Hospital, and her sister Bessie Lyons, Lady Superintendent at the Children's Hospital, Harcourt Street, trained at the Royal Southern Hospital in Liverpool. Both sisters were the daughters of a Westmeath gentleman and were described as 'genial and accomplished ladies, with the cordiality and happy manner of Irish country gentlewomen'.[77] Margaret Huxley, Lady Superintendent of Sir Patrick Dun's Hospital, was an English gentlewoman and the niece of the scientist Professor T. H. Huxley, and she received her certificate of training under Mrs Bedford Fenwick at St Bartholomew's Hospital in London.[78] Her successor, Miss Haughton, an English lady by birth and the niece of Professor Haughton of Trinity College, trained at Guy's Hospital, London. Miss Fullagar, Lady Superintendent of Mercer's Hospital and an Englishwoman of French Huguenot extraction, trained at Great Ormond Street and at the Clinical Infirmary, Manchester. Helena Bewley of the City of Dublin Hospital trained at the Doncaster General Infirmary. Helen Shuter, who succeeded Susan Beresford at the City of Dublin Hospital and who was described as a 'capable Englishwoman', trained at the Nightingale School at St Thomas's Hospital and at St Bartholomew's Hospital, and she held the post of sister-in-charge at St Thomas's.[79] Jane Eleanor Hughes, an Irish woman of Scottish and Welsh parentage and the first Lady Superintendent at the Whitworth Medical Hospital, received her diploma at the Brownlow Hill Hospital in Liverpool, one of the first hospitals outside of London to introduce the Nightingale reforms.[80] Miss Carson Rae, Lady Superintendent of Cork Street Fever Hospital, trained at the Westminster Hospital and was sister-in-charge and night superintendent at the Marylebone Infirmary.

Belonging to the same class as their employers, the lady superintendents held similar views to their employers on health and sanitation, morality and discipline, and the place of deference among the classes. They were also of the same class, religious denomination and ideological persuasion as their English counterparts; having received their nurse training in the reformed voluntary hospitals in England, it is unsurprising that they should take the Nightingale model as their model for nursing and sanitary reform.

The title 'Lady Superintendent' denoted that the holder of the office was a member of the middle or upper-middle class and that she held a position of authority with wide ranging responsibilities.[81] Because the position of lady superintendent was new to the hospital structure in Dublin, it required women of intelligence and strong will to ensure that the position as a senior and influential member of the hospital hierarchy would be consolidated. The establishment of a new nursing department with nursing divisions throughout the hospital's clinical departments and the projects of nursing and sanitary reform would succeed only

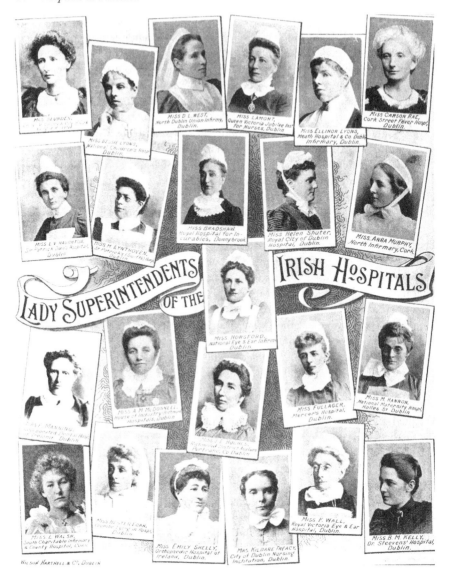

Figure 3.4 Lady Superintendents of Irish hospitals, 1904. Courtesy of the National Library of Ireland

if the lady superintendent could gain the confidence of the hospital board of management. With this confidence would come the sort of influence and autonomy needed to effect the required changes; in women like Helena Bewley, Susan Beresford, Eleanor Hughes and Annie McDonnell, the Dublin hospitals found the capable women to successfully complete the task in hand.

Sometimes referred to as 'Nightingale matrons', the first lady superintendents were true pioneers who had to front a world dominated by men and overcome prejudice against women, illness and poverty.[82] In reforming nursing and sanitation in the Dublin hospitals, their task was enormous. They were required to replace long established but outdated systems of care with an entirely new system that had been introduced only a few short years earlier in the prominent London hospitals. They were required to replace an entire untrained workforce with a new group of workers, for whose professional training they were also responsible. They were required to re-organize the hospital household and supervise its ancillary services, including laundry, dietary, and waste disposal. To introduce the changes, they had to enforce discipline, change attitudes and behaviour, sometimes face down resistance from established matrons, and engender respect for the authority of their new office. To make such profound changes that affected so many, often whole families, they needed not only the authorization of the hospital managers, but also the sort of authority and respect that could only come with the authority and respect that was conferred on their class.[83] They also derived much of their authority from the fact that they themselves were 'properly trained' in the new system of lady nursing, a system that was designed by and for their class.[84]

The lady superintendents were pioneers not only of hospital reform, but also of women's work and women's education and training at a time when training was not considered appropriate for women's professions, such as teaching and nursing.[85] Entering the public sphere through nursing provided middle-class women with opportunities that would otherwise have been closed to them, and the cut and thrust of life as a lady superintendent could give enormous personal and professional fulfilment. However, on entering the voluntary hospital, they had entered a male domain that could be alien and hostile.[86] In this domain, they afforded deference to the hospital administrator's administrative authority and to the clinician's clinical authority.[87]

Conclusions

On the evidence of the two case studies presented, it may be concluded that the story of the reform of nursing in the Dublin hospitals was the story of a fairly rapid transition from an old to a new order. The evidence indicates that by introducing probationership training as the central part of their project of reform, the Dublin hospitals achieved real and tangible improvements in the quality of patient care, in hospital sanitation, and in the general level of order within the hospital wards.

The reform of nursing in the Dublin hospitals is also a part of the story of the advancement of hospital scientific medicine, the consolidation of the hospital as the predominant model of organized healthcare delivery in Ireland, and the consolidation of medical hegemony through the institutionalization and control of nursing.[88] It is also a story of the advancement of middle and upper class values in a key area of social policy. Before the reforms, the day-to-day running of the hospital ward was largely in the hands of the uneducated poorer classes; by introducing lady superintendents and a 'better class' of nurse, the reforms resulted in a colonization of the hospital ward by the middle classes.

If the reforms represented the attainment of a new and respectable occupation for middle-class women, it is not certain that the final outcome of the project represented a net advancement in the cause of women, when one considers the plight of the untrained nurses and matrons, who were the principal casualties of the reforms. At a human level, one of the most striking features of the process of reform was the wave of dismissals that accompanied the introduction of the new system of nursing. In this way, the reforms touched directly the lives of ordinary women in profound ways. The fates of Bessie Fleming of the City of Dublin Hospital, of Julia Callery and Julia Hayden of the Richmond Hospital, and those of the untrained matrons Mrs Finlay and Mrs Byrne were decided in the demotions, dismissals and forced retirements that were an integral part of the reforms. These untrained nurses and their counterparts in the other Dublin hospitals were women whose circumstances were greatly altered in the transition from the old to the new system. Many had provided long and faithful service in the voluntary hospitals and some had doubtless developed considerable expertise.[89] Thus, while the reforms opened a new area of work for middle-class women, in doing so, it displaced many other women from the poorer class.

For Dublin's principal hospitals, the transition from the old to the new system of nursing was all but complete by about 1895. The nursing arrangements were transformed, and the training of nurses was an explicit activity. The probationer in training became an important material asset for the voluntary hospital. She provided relatively cheap labour in the hospital wards during her probationership training and was contractually obliged to give two years of service to the hospital when trained, and she generated much needed revenue, through the nursing of external private cases. For institutions like the City of Dublin Hospital and the Dublin House of Industry Hospitals, the new nursing arrangements provided an inexpensive, efficient and compliant workforce.[90] It is therefore unsurprising then that the transition to the new order should occur with such relative speed.

4 'Exemplary conduct and character'

The lady nurses of the Dublin hospitals

By the early the 1890s, the voluntary hospitals of Dublin had begun to experience the benefits that came with the improvements in hospital management, and nowhere were these benefits more apparent than in the hospitals' nursing arrangements and in hospital sanitation. The lady superintendents headed the nursing departments and reported directly to the boards of management as professionals in their own right. Trained nurses assisted by probationers in training provided skilled nursing care. Nurses experienced greatly improved conditions of employment, including increased salary, longer recreation periods, and comfortable living arrangements. Along with the transformation in nursing, the occupational status of the nurse was also transformed as a result of the reforms. By the mid-1890s, the movement to introduce lady nursing was viewed as a success, and was described as 'one of the swiftest and most remarkable of modern times'.[1]

In the 1890s, the curricular experiences of the first cohorts of young women who entered the new nurse training schemes in the Dublin voluntary hospitals were not unrelated to social developments occurring outside of the hospitals. Their curricular experiences occurred within the broader context of developments and activities related to the role of women and women's education in the late Victorian period. Moreover, the establishment of nursing as an essentially middle-class, secular-professional social practice was part of a wider process of social change in the late nineteenth century, and involving middle-class women and their role in society.

Women's education

When probationership training for nurses commenced in Dublin in the 1880s, it began at a time when a movement for equal educational provision for middle-class women was well advanced, and new opportunities for women in education were opening up. However, late Victorian beliefs concerning womanhood, women's education and the woman's role greatly restricted both the quantity and quality of educational provision for women. The preservation of male exclusivity in professions like medicine and the legal profession and the operation of guilds and apprenticeships restricted women's access to higher education and to areas of work that brought high status.[2] Another impediment was the attitude of many middle-class parents to the education of their daughters. The Schools Inquiry Commission of 1867–1868 reported on the 'general indifference of parents to girl's education, both in itself and as compared to that of boys', and pointed to the prejudice of many parents in relation to the education of their daughters, whereby girls were considered 'less capable of mental cultivation, and less in need of it, than boys'.[3] The sole desire of many middle-class parents was to see their daughters prepared for marriage.

The education of women was the subject of discourse in English writing from at least the early seventeenth century.[4] Arguments against higher education for women were predicated on extant theories concerning womanhood that ranged from scientific treatise on women's physical and mental inferiority to the view that education would render women incapable of performing their roles as wives and mothers.[5] Nineteenth-century middle-class constructions of womanhood involved a number of themes, including the emphasis on men's natural mental and physical superiority over women, the social dominance of men, and the threat to social order that any change in this status quo might represent.[6] In these constructions, a number of dyads were created, such as male strength–female frailty and male provider–female helpmate.[7] In 1887, the theorist George J. Romanes, treating on the mental differences between men and women, reasoned that, owing to the development of the brain, there was 'a greater power of amassing knowledge on the part of the male'.[8] The woman reader of the treatise might be consoled by the writer's assertion that women gained certain advantages over men in having a 'greater refinement of the sense organs', and in the fact that 'the meritorious qualities' of the female mind included affection, sympathy, devotion, self-denial, reverence, veneration, religious feeling and general morality. Higher education should take account of the mental differences between men and women and it should take account of the social position of women; it should 'keep the male and female types essentially different'.[9]

When set alongside views on the woman's physical and mental capacities to work and learn, the social construction of the woman's vocation – ascribed as wifehood, motherhood and home management – provided the grounds for determining and delimiting the sort of employment and educational provision available to women. Beliefs about the woman's place and theories of the woman's mental capacities did not merely limit the range of opportunities available to women in education, but also determined the social construction of the woman qua student and, consequentially, the sort of curriculum that she could experience.[10] The fundamental distinction between the education of men and women was the association of the former with public life and the latter with the home or private life.[11] On this basis, women's educational provision tended to take the form of special provision, i.e. education for women qua women; many middle-class young women attended private finishing schools, where they learned the social skills essential for the role of a 'lady'.[12] Especially prevalent among the upper middle classes, this type of education stressed training in 'accomplishments' related to feminine etiquette and decorum, and included training in vocational skills needed for work in the management of the home.[13] The curriculum for 'ladylike' women included reading, writing, arithmetic, English and the Bible, and practical classes in drawing, singing and botany.[14] In the view of Margaret Byers, the nineteenth-century Belfast campaigner for women's education, this curriculum was limited to subjects that could be displayed in the drawing room.[15]

In the face of strong opposition, a campaign for women's entry to higher education was conducted throughout the nineteenth century. Campaigners saw equal opportunities in education as the means of attaining sexual equality, and women's education was becoming increasingly associated with intellectual equality, vocational preparation, financial independence and, ultimately, with the development of the self.[16] The movement for the advancement of women's education aimed to challenge the notion that women did not need education, save that which made them better wives and mothers, and it aimed to promote women's access to institutes of education that were closed to them.[17]

In the second half of the nineteenth century, through economic necessity and a more liberal outlook on women's education, the cultivation of 'showy accomplishments' over the development of the intellect as the main function of women's education and the theory of men's superior intellectual capacity were being challenged.[18] Isabella Tod, one of the founders of the Belfast Ladies' Institute, complained that what was being taught to girls was simply 'the rudiments of those which form a portion of a boy's studies', and she called for higher education for women along the lines of a 'broad foundation in liberal studies'.[19] The campaign for women's education included calls for women's entry into the medical profession and the foremost campaigner in this area was Sophie Jex-Blake, who urged that equal facilities of study be afforded 'to all earnest students in connection with the national universities'.[20]

The campaign for women's education achieved some limited success, with the opening of Alexandra College in Dublin and Victoria College in Belfast.[21] Founded for middle-class Irish girls in 1866 by Anne Jellicoe and the Protestant Archbishop of Dublin Richard Chenevix Trench, Alexandra College was modelled on Queen's College, Harley Street in London, the first higher education college for women in England.[22] Alexandra College provided a broad curriculum of liberal studies at university level in subjects that included Latin, English, French, history, arithmetic, algebra and geometry, and it prepared future women teachers of these academic subjects; distinguished professors from Trinity College Dublin gave the lectures and set the examinations.[23] It was only after 1879, with the passage of the University Bill for Ireland, that women began to gain a tenuous foothold in higher education and in 1904 Trinity College opened its degrees to women.[24]

In the last two decades of the nineteenth century, employment opportunities were increasingly available to young middle-class women, especially in the civil service.[25] However, in gaining access to professional and white-collar work, women were obtaining positions that were held to be female domain activities. Typing was likened to piano playing and clerical work drew on women's toleration of repetition, while teaching and nursing were an extension of women's nurturing.[26] However, as girls successfully competed with boys for employment in clerical work, their secondary education became more similar to that of boys.[27] Only with the passage of the Universities Act of 1908 and the establishment of the National University could women be assured of higher education that was de jure if not de facto similar to that of men.

Apprenticeship nurse training

The movement for the advancement of women's higher education bore a number of striking similarities with the movement for nursing reform in Dublin. Both movements occurred in and around the same period in the nineteenth century, and the principal campaigners in both were Protestant middle-class women and influential professional men. While she was not a member of the important decision making body of Alexandra College, the College Council, Anne Jellicoe achieved great success in advancing higher education for women by establishing strategic alliances with men of influence, including influential educationalists from Trinity College.[28] Her counterpart in nursing, the lady superintendent, established strategic alliances with influential medical men. Jellicoe held the title of Lady Superintendent at Alexandra College; in this role her duties included being responsible for order and discipline within the college, including the supervision of the servants, taking charge of the library, and keeping the daily accounts.[29] Like her nursing counterpart, Jellicoe was concerned with the better education and advancement of gentlewomen, and she opened up new opportunities for women of her class to enter the domain of professional work.

When nursing reformers in Dublin introduced the new training schemes for lady nurses, they too were introducing a new way for women to enter into paid professional work. However, unlike the curriculum at Alexandra College, probationership nurse training was regarded less as a new form of higher education and more a new sphere of employment for educated ladies.[30] In consequence of this view, apprenticeship nurse training did not have the status of a *higher* education, but was a vocational extension of secondary education. It was a form of vocational-professional training that combined technical instruction with elements of the curriculum for young ladies; having features of the finishing school for young ladies, apprenticeship nurse training has been likened to the girls' domestic academy model of education.[31] As such, it contained many elements that reflected late nineteenth-century views on the sort of a curriculum that was deemed appropriate for young ladies and, like the finishing school, the nursing school represented a form of *special* educational provision; it was an education for women qua women.

The faults of the untrained hospital nurse, including her alleged misconduct, were seen more in terms of the poor moral character of the lower class and less in terms of poor technical skills.[32] Thus, aside from its role of providing a skilled medical auxiliary, nurse training should also promote the development of the nurse's moral character. The Nightingale model of nurse training was designed for this dual purpose and it was the model with which the new lady superintendents of the Dublin hospitals were familiar when they embarked on their reforms in the 1880s. A secular-professional model that was premised on the recruit being a carefully selected Christian, it would develop the nurse's character through disciplined work and submission to authority and, through apprenticeship training, it would develop her technical proficiency.[33] As a model of character training, it was imbibed with both religious and secular influences in English public life; in Nightingale's writings and in the attitudes of the Nightingale matrons in the London hospitals, character formation – demonstrated as kindness, conscientiousness, obedience and loyalty – was what mattered in the training of lady nurses.[34] Training was aimed at 'virtuous womanhood' and, while it prepared the nurse for her role in the hospital and in private nursing, its *academic* function in this regard was somewhat redundant, given the fact that many Nightingale matrons were ambivalent about theoretical education and development of the intellect and were disdainful of academic cleverness.[35]

The Nightingale model drew much of its influence from the denominational tradition of sick nursing, such as that proffered by Anglican sisterhoods, the Lutheran Deaconess movement in Germany, and the Catholic Sisters of Mercy.[36] In a more obvious way, it also drew its influence from the St John's House model of nurse training, which Robert Bentley Todd established in London in 1848. St John's House was an Anglican sisterhood that spearheaded nursing reform in England, providing modern nursing services to a number of the London hospitals.[37] The St John's House model was based on the moral and social development of the nurse through discipline and social control within apprenticeship training.[38]

Through the recruitment of a better class of nurse, the Nightingale model of reform also reconstructed the class basis of nursing.[39] While the recruitment of a better class of nurse would in itself greatly improve the nurse's moral character, it seems that the system of training would leave nothing to chance, and the training regime appeared to pay particular attention to its remit of character development. In the course of her training, the nurse's character would be fashioned out of a pedagogical experience that emphasized disciplined work, custodial control and obedience to authority. The lady nurse experienced a highly regulated and structured regime, having congregational-like features, in areas such as nurses' dining, recreation, and hours of duty. Nurse training became a process of disciplinary training of the type that was already in place in schools and factories and, in common with these settings, it had surveillance features and functions.[40] The lady superintendent strictly controlled the probationer's work during her working day and, while off duty, the home sister supervised her recreation in the nurses' homes.[41] The nurses' home was an expression of the wider concern in Victorian society to ensure regularity, order, decency and the segregation of the sexes.[42] Unlike halls of residence in universities, which functioned to provide a place of study and solitude, the nurses' home functioned more as a place of confinement and surveillance, and the total regime of control secured the probationer's deferential and disciplined labour.[43]

New training schemes

By the early 1890s, nurse training schemes based on the Nightingale model had been established in all of the major voluntary hospitals in Dublin, including the hospitals founded and/or managed by Catholic religious congregations, and at the new training institutes, such as the City of Dublin Nurses Training Institution. While a training school for nurses was established at the Adelaide Hospital in 1858, at the time that the Nursing Committee of the Dublin Hospital Sunday Fund made its enquiries in 1879, nurse training was not being conducted at that hospital. It is therefore probable that the first school to offer formal and systematic nurse training in Dublin was the Dublin Nurses' Training Institution, located at No. 4 Holles Street. The Institution was founded in 1866 by the Protestant Archbishop of Dublin Richard Chenevix Trench as an independent institute for the training of Protestant nurses.[44] For periods between 1867 and 1883, the Dublin Nurses Training Institution entered into arrangements for the training of probationers, initially with Dr Steevens' Hospital and later with Sir Patrick Dun's Hospital.[45] The arrangement between Dr Steevens' Hospital and the Institution meant that the Dr Steevens' Hospital was the first hospital in Dublin to receive nurses for training in its wards.[46] Both Dr Steevens' and Sir Patrick Dun's hospitals established their own nurse training schools in 1879 and 1883 respectively.

Located at 101 St Stephen's Green, St Patrick's Home was established in 1876 for the purpose of 'supplying trained nurses to the sick poor in their own homes' and was affiliated with the Queen's Institute of District Nursing.[47] The City of Dublin Nursing Institution provided probationership training in association with the City of Dublin Hospital between 1883 and 1900, after which time the latter institution operated its own nursing school.[48] The City of Dublin Nursing Institution also had an arrangement with Mercer's Hospital for the supply of trained nurses. Bearing the same name as the training institution at Holles Street, the Dublin Nurses' Training Institution at No. 26 Usher's Quay was founded by Mrs Eliza Browne in 1882 and had an arrangement with Dr Steevens' Hospital for the clinical instruction of probationers.[49] In 1884, the Dublin Red Cross Nursing Sisters established a House and Training School for Nurses at 87 Harcourt Street and the probationers of the Red Cross received their practical training at the National Children's Hospital, Harcourt Street, and at the Meath Hospital and County Infirmary at Heytesbury Street.[50]

Arrangements for the systematic training of probationers at the Dublin House of Industry Hospitals were established in 1890. After 1894, the Dublin House of Industry Hospitals, Sir Patrick Dun's Hospital, Dr Steevens' Hospital, the Nurses' Training Institution at Usher's Quay, and the Dublin Orthopaedic Hospital were affiliated to the Dublin Metropolitan Technical School for Nurses, a centralized training school that provided a programme of systematic teaching and uniform examinations for the probationers of its affiliated hospitals.[51]

Following the recommendations of the Dublin Hospitals Commission of 1887, the Sisters of Mercy established training schools for lay probationers at the

Charitable Infirmary and the Mater Misericordiae Hospital in 1891. A training school for lay probationers was established at St Vincent's Hospital in 1892. Elsewhere in Ireland in the early 1890s, schools of nursing were operating at both the North Infirmary and the South Infirmary in Cork, at the Women's and Children's Hospital, Cork, and at Barrington's Hospital in Limerick. In the 1890s in all but two counties of Ireland, Westmeath and Carlow, nurse training schools were receiving probationers, and at least fifty-two hospitals throughout the country were offering nurse training.[52]

With all of the major voluntary hospitals operating apprenticeship-training schemes for lady nurses by 1895, common features of probationership training were evident across all hospitals; the lady nurses in the Dublin hospitals shared common experiences in relation to recruitment and selection, conditions of employment, pedagogy, and work and recreation.

Recruitment and selection and conditions of employment

The requirement that prospective candidates for probationership training be well educated, of good character, and pay a relatively substantial entry fee indicates that well-to-do families provided the recruitment ground for probationers. The lady nurses of the Dublin hospitals were recruited from Dublin and the provinces and from a spectrum of Victorian social strata that included the lower-middle class, better-off artisans and farmers, and the well-placed families of the middle and upper-middle classes.[53]

Many hospitals operated a dual system of 'ordinary' probationer and 'paying' probationer. This two-tier system originated at St John's House in London and it was also in place at the Nightingale School at St Thomas's Hospital, where the paying probationer had prestige and privileges over her ordinary counterpart.[54] Paying probationers paid a substantial entry fee and received no salary. It is therefore probable that they were drawn from the wealthier families of the recruits to nursing and that ordinary probationers were recruited from the artisan and lower-middle classes. The paying probationer enjoyed a more favourable contract of employment, including a shorter training period and, while learning the skills of sick nursing, was groomed to assume a leadership role in nursing; the ordinary probationer was trained for the work of sick nursing. The dual probationership system operated in many of the Dublin hospitals, including the City of Dublin Hospital, Dr Steevens' Hospital, and the Dublin House of Industry Hospitals. The regulations for probationers at the Dublin House of Industry Hospitals included a description of the system:

> Candidates are of two classes – the first paying £30 for one year's training; the second binding themselves to the Hospitals, but paying no fee ... Candidates belonging to the first class receive no salary. Those belonging to the second class will be paid as follows: – First year ... £10 per annum ... Second year ... £12 per annum, Third year ... £14 per annum.[55]

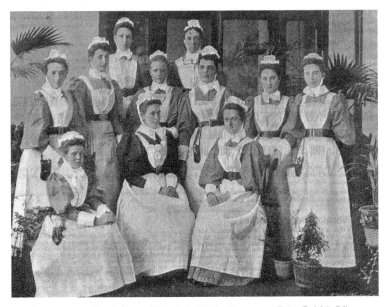

Figure 4.1 Lady nurses, Jervis Street Hospital, 1895. Courtesy of the British Library

The probationary period at the Dublin House of Industry Hospitals was three months, but the Lady Superintendent could dispense with the services of the probationer after one month's trial, and probationers were required to give their services either to the hospital or in private service. Probationers received a uniform, lodging and boarding and, upon passing the examination at the end of the first year, received a certificate of competence. Paying probationers were permitted to leave after one year. The House and Training School for Nurses established by the Dublin Red Cross Nursing Sisters at Harcourt Street recruited exclusively from the upper classes, where probationers paid an entry fee of fifty guineas, enjoyed a separate room, and were described as 'gentlewomen by birth and social position'.[56]

Intending probationers at the Dublin Metropolitan Technical School for Nurses were required to pass a preliminary examination in reading, spelling, writing and arithmetic, 'corresponding to the fourth class of National Education'.[57] Candidates applying to the Adelaide Hospital were expected to be 'fairly well educated (under which head marked attention … [was] expected to the item of reading aloud)'.[58] Candidates seeking admission to nurse training at the Royal Hospital for Incurables at Donnybrook were expected to be 'active, industrious, thoroughly trustworthy…and [be] able to read and write well'.[59] At the Mater Misericordiae Hospital, candidates for probationership training were required to be 'not only well educated, but well recommended and of good social status'.[60] When the Irish Sisters of Charity commenced the training of lay nurses at St Vincent's Hospital in 1892, Mother Canisius Cullen was said to have had the good fortune to find 'a cultured gentlewoman, who … fixed the standard for the Nursing School'.[61]

The entry fee for probationership training in the 1890s was typically £10 in most of the Dublin voluntary hospitals. The City of Dublin Nursing Institution charged a fee of thirty guineas, while the lady nurses of the Red Cross attached to the Meath Hospital paid a fee of fifty guineas, which also gave them membership of the Red Cross Order.[62] While most training hospitals charged an entry fee, a salary of approximately £10 per annum was also paid, usually at the commencement of training or upon completion of the first year of training, with incremental annual increases, usually of £2, during subsequent years.

The minimum age of entry to training differed among the various hospitals and training institutions. At the City of Dublin Nursing Institution and the Charitable Infirmary, the minimum age of entry was twenty years, at St Vincent's Hospital it was twenty-one years, and at Sir Patrick Dun's, Dr Steevens' and the Adelaide hospitals it was twenty-three years.[63] Where it was specified, the upper age limit ranged from thirty years (Sir Patrick Dun's Hospital) to forty years (City of Dublin Nursing Institution). Candidates applying for entry to Dr Steevens' Hospital were required to be 'in good health, of average height and physique, well educated, and of an age from 23 to 35 years'.[64] The Mater Misericordiae Hospital favoured 'mature girls in their mid-twenties, who could bring with them a good education, work experience and a maturity that would contribute to the standard of nursing care'.[65]

Recruitment of probationers was conducted on the basis of a written application to the lady superintendent. Selection was based on a personal interview with the lady superintendent, followed by approval by the hospital board of

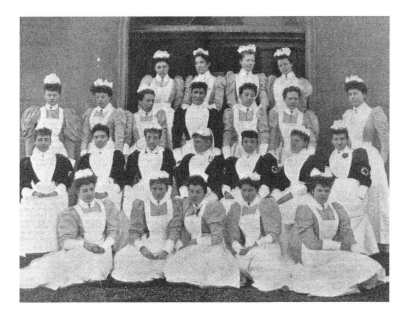

Figure 4.2 'Ladies by birth and social position', lady nurses of the Red Cross Order, 1895.
Courtesy of the British Library

management, and candidates were required to present letters of recommenda-tion. Candidates applying to the Red Cross Order were required to present three letters of recommendation from a medical man, a clergyman, and an inti-mate personal friend. Similarly, at the Charitable Infirmary, intending probationers applied to the Matron for the necessary entrance papers and were required to produce testimonials of character. Selection at St Vincent's Hospital was made on the basis of a personal interview with the Superioress and two character references.

Candidates entering probationership training were required to undertake a trial term, usually of three months' duration. At the Dublin House of Industry Hospitals, the lady superintendent could dismiss a pupil at the end of the first month 'in cases of marked unsuitability for the nursing profession'.[66] At the Dublin Nurses' Training Institution at Usher's Quay, after the trial period of one month, probationers who were 'well fitted by their intelligence, sound constitution and aptitude for the nursing profession' were accepted for training.[67] A one-month's 'preliminary trial' period also operated at St Vincent's Hospital, during which time 'if the pupil's health or powers of adaptability for the nursing profes-sion be found to be insufficient, she shall be released from her intended engagement'.[68] Dismissal after this initial preliminary trial period was also possi-ble at St Vincent's Hospital:

> at all times during the nurse's training and subsequent career on the staff of the hospital it must be understood that the Superioress holds the power of instant dismissal in the case of any neglect of duty or fault in personal con-duct.[69]

Aside from the trial period, the duration of probationership training at most of the Dublin hospitals was one year. A diploma or a certificate of training was awarded at end of this period. Training institutions like the Dublin Metropolitan Technical School for Nurses and the Dublin Nurses' Training Institution awarded a diploma, denoting the successful completion of *theoretical* instruction, while the probationer's training hospital awarded a separate certificate of training, denot-ing the successful completion of *practical* instruction in the hospital wards.

With the exception of paying probationers, most of the lady nurses of the Dublin hospitals were required to provide three years of service following the ini-tial one-year training period. However, paying probationers were encouraged to remain in the service of their training hospital after the one-year training period.

Instruction

The lady nurses of the Dublin hospitals received instruction from medical men and from the lady superintendent in subjects related to hospital medicine and sick nursing. The instruction given to probationers at the Mater Misericordiae Hospital consisted of courses in anatomy, physiology, hygiene, and medical, surgical and gynaecological nursing given by surgeons and doctors at the Hospital. The Matron

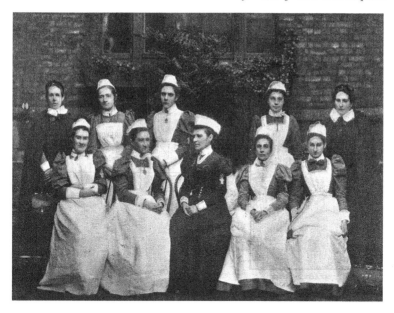

Figure 4.3 Lady nurses, St Patrick's Home, Dublin, 1895. Courtesy of the British Library

Miss McGivney lectured on invalid cookery, ward work and general nursing, and instructed probationers in the management of fever cases, the skills of treating with poultices, fomentations, leeches, dry cupping, applying ice bags, and the technique of giving medicines, powders and pills.[70] Miss McGivney, who trained at the London Hospital, was described as a quiet, refined and helpful person and was reputed to have been an excellent teacher, spending time on the wards with the probationers.[71] At the City of Dublin Nursing Institution, probationers received instruction in anatomy and physiology from visiting medical staff of the City of Dublin Hospital, and the lady superintendent gave instruction in hygiene, general nursing, and the nursing of medical, surgical and ophthalmic cases. At the Dublin Metropolitan Technical School for Nurses, probationers attended for three terms and received lectures in elementary anatomy and surgical anatomy, physiology and the administration of drugs, and hygiene and invalid cookery.

During training, probationers provided the nursing care in the hospital wards, where they were expected to develop their nursing skills. They were placed on a rotational basis in the various clinical departments of the hospital for periods of six to eight weeks. It was understood that affording probationers the opportunities to gain the widest possible range of practical experience in a variety of clinical departments was necessary for the development of proficiency. While working on the wards, probationers received instruction from the lady superintendent and acted under the direction of the certified nurse.

Examinations in theoretical and clinical instruction were part of the curricular experiences of the lady nurses of the Dublin hospitals in the 1890s. Examinations

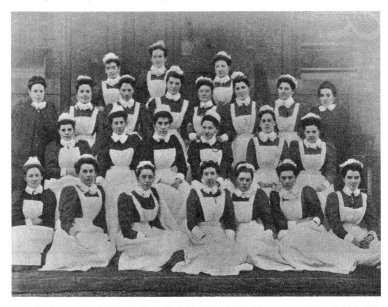

Figure 4.4 Lady nurses, Adelaide Hospital, Dublin, 1895. Courtesy of the British Library

were conducted by medical men and by the lady superintendent, and served both educational and administrative functions related to progression through training and eligibility for the awarding of a certificate of training. Upon completion of one year of training at the City of Dublin Nursing Institution, probationers were required to present themselves for examination before the Examining Board; doctors Boyd, Kidd and Harley were listed as the examiners in 1894.[72] At the Dublin Metropolitan Technical Schools for Nurses, probationers were examined at the end of each term and their names were arranged 'in order of merit in answering' and, in the case of a probationer failing an examination, she was permitted to re-present on payment of a fee.[73]

Recreation

Probationers' duty times and their off-duty arrangements were highly regulated. At many hospitals, including Sir Patrick Dun's, the City of Dublin, the Meath and Mercer's, the hours of duty were from 7 am to 9 pm and most hospitals permitted half an hour for each meal break. However, the arrangements for nurses' recreation varied among the hospitals. At Sir Patrick Dun's Hospital, nurses were permitted off duty on two days per week at 4 pm. At the City of Dublin Hospital, the recreation time was daily from 3 pm to 5 pm or from 5.30 pm to 9 pm. Dr Steevens' Hospital permitted three hours' recreation on alternative days. Most hospitals granted one month of annual holidays.

Probationers were provided with four meals a day that included breakfast, dinner, tea, and supper, and the lady superintendent or the matron supervised

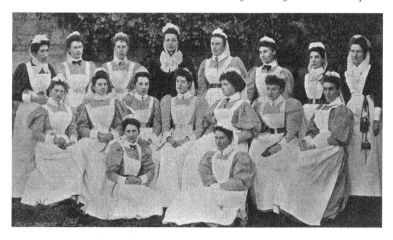

Figure 4.5 Lady nurses, South Infirmary, Cork, 1896. Courtesy of the British Library

probationers during mealtimes. Residential accommodation was provided within the new nurses' homes that were developed as part of the nursing reforms, and living arrangements generally consisted of a room or dormitory, board and washing. The nurses and probationers at the Mater Misericordiae Hospital were provided with a comfortable home at Nos. 32 and 35 Eccles Street. The probationers of the Red Cross Order resided at the Home in Harcourt Street, where each lady nurse had a separate room. The living arrangements at the Charitable Infirmary were described in 1895 as follows:

> Nurses and Probationers are at present lodged in the hospital, where they have commodious dormitories, and enjoy a cheerful sitting-room, provided with a piano, where they practice (sic) music or needle-work and read during their hours of recreation.[74]

Miss Gabrielle Tierney presided over probationers' domestic arrangements at the Dublin Nurses' Training Institution at Usher's Quay. While off duty in the nurses' home, probationers were subject to Miss Tierney's authority and she was empowered to dismiss a probationer for breach of duty, and each probationer was expected to keep her own room 'in perfect order'.

While living arrangements and recreational amenities were favourable, restrictions were imposed on probationers during their off-duty time. In consequence, probationers experienced a regime that was congregational and custodial. At the Dublin Nurses' Training Institution, probationers were not permitted to absent themselves from the nurses' home in the evening, unless with special permission. Nurses residing at the nurses' home of the City of Dublin Nursing Institution at 27 Upper Baggot Street were under the authority of its Lady Manager, who arranged their home comforts and granted them leave of absence when required. When absent on recreation, probationers of the Red Cross Order were expected to return to the home at 5 pm, but for 'special purposes' and on application to the lady superintendent, were granted leave of absence until 9.15 pm. These same probationers were expected to attend public worship, to observe strict punctuality at meals, and to render 'explicit obedience to the orders of the Lady Superintendent and housekeeper'.[75]

A description of a day in the life of the probationer at the Adelaide Hospital in 1895 indicates that the overall pattern of her day was highly structured:

> The hours of duty for Probationers and trained nurses in hospital is 87 hours per week, and the terms are adjusted so as to come lightly on the workers. The dinner hour may vary. There are two half-holidays in the week, from 3 o'clock to 9 pm; and on Sunday alternately, from 11 am to 2 pm, and from 3 till 9 pm with an additional hour and a half for rest or recreation on four days of the week … Nurses going on day duty are called at 6 am, and get tea or coffee, with bread and butter, before they enter the wards; they have breakfast, with meat or eggs, at 8.30; a luncheon of milk and bread and butter in the ward kitchen at 11 o'clock and dinner is served in the dining-hall, presided over by the matron, assistant matron and divisional nurses, from 1.30 to 2.15 pm.; five o'clock tea is prepared in the ward kitchens … and a meat supper is laid in the dining hall at 9 pm.[76]

The lady nurses of the Red Cross Order also experienced a highly structured day:

> Probationers breakfast at 7 am, sisters at 9.30; dinner is served at 1.30 pm, tea at 6, and supper at 9 pm. All retire to rest at 10 pm, and lights are extinguished at 11.[77]

While the life of the probationer was highly regulated, recreation was encouraged. At the Charitable Infirmary, probationers were 'in *all* domestic matters under the authority of the Sisters, who are most considerate of the home comforts of their inmates, while their amusements and recreation is by no means curtailed'.[78] At Cork Street Fever Hospital, recreation was considered to be essential for the health and rejuvenation of the probationers:

> One whole day is allowed in each month, and a continuous fortnight, which may be extended to three weeks by special order, is granted once in each year. The Leave of nurses is given for their recreation and health, and consequently for the benefit of good nursing of the patients.[79]

At this same hospital, 'every attention' was paid to the regulation of the probationers' recreation and nothing was permitted to interfere with it. However, for probationers in some institutions, the protection of their recreation time could not always be guaranteed. At the Mater Misericordiae Hospital, nurses who were resident in the nurses' home at Eccles Street were expected to attend in the wards of the hospital, should the sister require their services. Recreation consisted of such

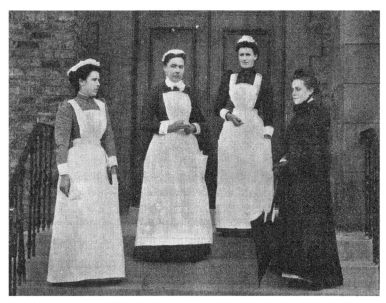

Figure 4.6 Indoor and outdoor uniform, Sir Patrick Dun's Hospital, 1895 (Miss Huxley is second from left). Courtesy of the British Library

activities as reading, music and needlework. As recreational activities, needlework and sewing were especially important, and it appears that a number of institutions used this activity to their advantage; at St Vincent's Hospital, nurses were expected to 'willingly assist in needlework' when off duty, while at the Charitable Infirmary, nurses when off duty were 'expected to assist in plain sewing or other duties required of them'.[80]

For the lady nurses of the Dublin hospitals in the 1890s, strict rules applied in relation to the consumption of alcohol. At the City of Dublin Nursing Institution, probationers were permitted 'no stimulants whatever … unless with special permission of a medical adviser', while at St Vincent's Hospital, no nurse or pupil was permitted to 'ask for or procure alcoholic stimulants of any kind … without the express recommendation of a medical attendant'.[81] When nursing private cases, nurses from the Dublin Nurses Training Institution were not permitted to procure, or accept when offered, either wine or spirits. Strict rules regarding the consumption of alcohol ensured that the probationer was capable of working and that she maintained the desired public image of respectability and decorum. The receiving of gratuities from patients was also prohibited.

'Lace-edge strings'

The nurse's uniform was the most visible expression of nursing reform and its distinctiveness indicated that the new lady nurses had arrived in the Dublin hospitals. The uniform symbolized the new status of the nurse as a professional health worker. Its predominantly white appearance was a metaphor for the new system of lady nursing, distinguishing it from the discredited former system proffered by untrained nurses, and the uniform was clearly intended to differentiate the lady nurse from other workers, most especially the untrained nurse and the domestic servant.[82]

Uniforms were of two principal types, namely indoor and outdoor. The indoor uniform was worn when on ward duty, while the outdoor uniform was worn when off duty. Probationers at Sir Patrick Dun's Hospital wore an outdoor uniform of dark green cloak with capes and a small straw bonnet. At the City of Dublin Nursing Institution, probationers were expected to wear the outdoor uniform at all times, save when on leave. The Adelaide nurse's indoor uniform was described as a 'dress of hail spot cotton print, white cap and apron, and small straw bonnet trimmed in blue, with cape-fronted cloak of blue cloth'.[83] The indoor uniform of the Royal Hospital for Incurables was 'of a pink zephyr, with linen aprons and the "Sister Dora" cap', while the outdoor uniform consisted of 'an olive green cloak, of thick cloth, made with full, loose cape to below the waist, and small bonnet trimmed with velvet to match'.[84] The indoor and outdoor uniforms for probationers at the Charitable Infirmary were described in 1895 as follows:

> The indoor uniform at Jervis Street is one of the prettiest among our many hospitals – a fresh cool, bright shade of sky-like blue, with a crossbar pattern of silky white upon it. The aprons are, of course, wide, with strapped bibs and large pockets, while the caps of thick white muslin, with lace edging, are varied by lace-edge strings for qualified nurses. The outdoor uniform is a long cloak of deep violet colour, shaped at the back, and having side capes to below the waist, with small straw bonnet trimmed in velvet to match the cloak.[85]

The nurse's uniform had features that distinguished the probationer and the trained nurse:

> The uniform [of the Dublin Nurses' Training Institution] is of blue striped Galtea, with full cascered, black cloak and small straw bonnet with long black gauze veil for out of doors; and wide linen aprons with pockets and the soft white caps are similar to those universally worn by the profession, and, is as also usual, the addition of strings marks the qualified nurse from the probationer.[86]

The nurse's uniform presented the public with an idealized image of gentlewomen, fittingly attired for their new role in the care of the sick in the reformed hospital wards.[87] Aside from its practical use, although this may be questionable, the uniform was an outward expression to the public at large that nursing was to be recognized as a respectable and responsible occupation and a distinct form of employment for gentlewomen.[88] The uniform was evidently an attractive garment in the late Victorian period, its design tending to mirror prevailing fashions in clothing.[89] Nevertheless, it functioned primarily as working apparel, designed to maintain hygiene and reduce the spread of contagion. The apron was also part of the nurse's uniform – probationers were usually supplied with up to twelve aprons – and it was intended to protect the main garment from organic fluids and household spillages.

The uniform was to be worn with no additional decorations or jewellery. The lady nurses of the Red Cross Order were permitted no trinkets, save 'a surgical chatelaine, containing scissors, spatula, etc., necessary to their ward work', while probationers at the Adelaide Hospital was expected to maintain 'an orderly, unostentatious style of dress'.[90] The indoor and outdoor uniforms, along with the rules governing how they were to be worn and the manner in which the nurse was expected to present herself in public, symbolized the control that was placed on the life of the probationer. The uniform also presented an image of the nurse as virtuous and upright, the bearer and the custodian of propriety and order. It became associated with cleanliness and hygiene, and the reformed, uniformed nurse embodied and, at the same time, consolidated in the public mind the image of the physically and morally clean nurse.[91] While designed to convey probity, purity and moral propriety and to serve as an instrument of control, paradoxically, the uniform may have had the opposite effect by promoting women's sexuality. The vivid descriptions of the 'prettiest' dresses, aprons and bonnets clearly, if inadvertently, conveyed powerful images of femininity.

'That highest walk of woman's work'

Along with transforming the quality of sick nursing care, the reform of nursing also greatly altered the public image of the nurse, and nursing was no longer viewed as a dubious occupation. As employment of 'the strictest decency, cleanliness, and

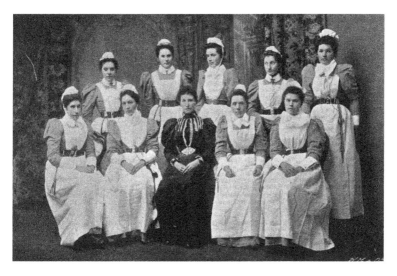

Figure 4.7 Lady nurses, Dublin Nurses' Training Institution, Usher's Quay, 1896. Courtesy of the British Library

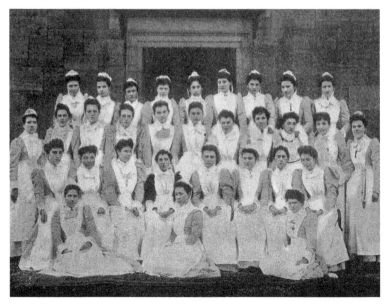

Figure 4.8 Lady nurses, Mater Misericordiae Hospital, 1895. Courtesy of the British Library

morality', nursing was promoted as a worthy occupation for educated gentle-women.[92] By the mid-1890s, when the reform of hospital nursing in Dublin was all but complete, sick nursing was held to be 'one of the most laudable undertakings … [and] that highest walk of woman's work'.[93]

While the introduction of lady nursing reconstructed the class basis of sick nursing, the two-tier 'ordinary' and 'paying' probationership system carried the class divisions of the period into the new system of nurse training and, far from creating a homogenous class, the two-tier system guarded the class divisions for the elite nursing leaders.[94] Many trained nurses, most especially the paying proba-tioners, were appointed to responsible and senior positions, reflecting the fact that lady nursing was a gateway to a respected professional career for gentlewomen. For many paying probationers, elevation to a senior position was rapid and a few, including Margaret Huxley, were appointed to the position of lady superinten-dent immediately upon completion of their training. Within a decade after the opening of the City of Dublin Nursing Institution, many of its trained nurses were appointed to the post of ward sister at the City of Dublin Hospital, and eight became matrons of hospitals.[95] Of the first cohort of sixteen probationers who entered training at the Mater Misericordiae Hospital in 1891, all took up respon-sible positions as nurses and three went on to become matrons.[96]

By the end of the nineteenth century, sick nursing in Ireland had attained a social standing and a respectability that would have been unthinkable at the time when the movement for nursing reform began in the early 1880s, and the terms 'profession' and 'nursing profession' were in common usage in popular discourse concerned with nursing. During the royal visit to Dublin in 1900, the matrons of the Dublin hospitals were presented to Queen Victoria at the Vice Regal Lodge. Led by Margaret Huxley, the matrons presented an address of welcome to the Queen and expressed their gratitude to her for her interest in promoting nurse training.[97] In a 'tribute to Dublin nursing' published in the society journal *The Lady of the House* in 1897, the writer Mary Costello praised the nurses who received their training under the lady nursing movement for their valuable work among the rich and poor:

> to be a perfect nurse means that both head and heart are stocked with some of the best things that nature has in her gift. For instance, not only with patience with the irritable and exacting, tenderness with the harsh and untender, but also with courage, firmness, intelligence and deftness.[98]

The writer remarked that skilled hospital training had resulted in a 'nice balancing of the faculties' and she highlighted the relationship of good nursing with feminine qualities, observing that 'with most good women, nursing is an instinct, fed … from the great maternal artery'. The introduction of lady nursing in Dublin had resulted in a great social gain, and just as the social reformers had intended, the trained nurse was capable of bringing order where there was disorder, cleanliness where there was dirt, and an end to disease. According to Costello, skilled hospital training had led to the successful eradication of a 'dirtborn plague' on the Island of Inniskea in the west of Ireland, and this fact showed 'what a salutary moral factor society has in the educated nurse when her heart is in her work'.[99]

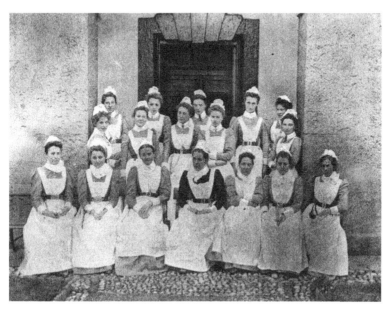

Figure 4.9 Lady nurses, Dr Steevens' Hospital, Dublin. Courtesy of the National Library of Ireland

Conclusions

When social reformers in Dublin introduced probationership nurse training, they were not introducing a new form of higher education for middle-class women, but were providing them with a means of entry to paid professional employment. As a female occupation, nursing exemplified gendered work and, from its inception as a social practice, the training of nurses also exemplified gendered education.[100] As with the mainstream of women's education in the late nineteenth century, constructions of womanhood, specifically those concerned with women's relationships with men, women as workers, and women's education, determined the curricular experiences of the first lady nurses of the Dublin hospitals. In this way, the pedagogic experience was derived not merely from the perspective of the probationer's training needs qua hospital nurse, but also from the perspective of her education needs qua woman.

While she worked and recreated, the probationer in the Dublin hospital experienced a highly regulated life, maintained through strict rules that governed her conduct and maintained surveillance over her. In imposing such an apparently restrictive regime, hospital authorities were preparing a nurse who could meet the demands of scientific medicine, and they were reflecting the prevailing demands of Victorian respectability and the time-oriented discipline of an industrialized society.[101] The nurse was expected to function in an unpredictable clinical environment, where the condition of acutely ill patients could change rapidly and, for this reason, she needed to be self-disciplined in her work, operating within the clear parameters of her clinical jurisdiction.

While the social movement that introduced lady nursing greatly altered the social status of nursing, the nurse was still both a woman and a doctor's assistant. She lived out these roles in a late Victorian society that was hierarchically structured along the lines of social class and gender. These same roles would continue to determine the content of her curricular experiences and would delimit the extent to which nursing could advance along a path towards higher education and the ranks of the learned professions. The subsequent expansion of nurse training in the early twentieth century coincided with a period of enormous change for women, a period which was characterized by the theme of 'modernity'.[102] This period was represented by the suffragist movement, by greater opportunities for women in employment and education and by what Lorentzon refers to as 'a greater spirit of female independence'.[103] This spirit of female independence would be expressed in the new crusade for nursing, the pursuit of professional regulation through state registration.

5 Professional regulation and the General Nursing Council for Ireland

While the movement for nursing reform in Ireland was viewed as a success in having greatly improved the quality of sick nursing, for many nursing leaders, the process of reform was not yet complete. No sooner had the system of lady nursing been introduced than a new phase of nursing reform was commencing. Begun in the last decade of the nineteenth century, this new phase of reform was aimed at attaining professional regulation, through state registration and the standardization of nurse training. While it was an international endeavour, the campaign for professional regulation of nursing was also conducted in Ireland. A protracted campaign lasting for more than two decades, it achieved its ultimate goal of registration legislation with the enactment of the Nurses' Registration (Ireland) Act in 1919.[1]

The nursing cause

The campaign for state registration, referred to as the 'nursing cause', was conducted by a cadre of elite nursing leaders and by nursing's new professional bodies, including the British Nurses' Association and the Irish Nurses' Association. Doctors, hospital administrators, and Members of Parliament were also involved.[2] The subject of extensive research by nurse historians, the campaign has been described as a conflict between opposing factions involved in a divisive struggle lasting for some thirty years and involving principles, vested interests and personal quarrels.[3]

The principal protagonists in the early years of the campaign included Florence Nightingale, who opposed state registration, and Ethel Bedford Fenwick, who vigorously pursued it. In Ireland, the most prominent activist in the pursuit of the nursing cause was Margaret Huxley, Matron of Sir Patrick Dun's Hospital and a close friend and professional ally of Mrs Bedford Fenwick[4] The proponents of state regulation wanted to ensure that, through registration legislation, only properly trained nurses from approved hospitals would be permitted to practise as a nurse. A regulated nursing workforce would protect the public from incompetent and unsafe nurses. In evidence to the House of Commons Select Committee on the Registration of Nurses in 1904, Margaret Huxley declared: 'if you do not educate your nurse, in the end the public must suffer'.[5] The campaign envisaged the establishment of a central nursing council to oversee standards of entry and training and to establish uniform examinations and certification.[6]

Mrs Ethel Bedford Fenwick was the leader of the campaign in England. Appointed Matron of St Bartholomew's Hospital in London in 1881 at age twenty-four, she was the wife of Dr Bedford Fenwick, then a prominent London physician and also a strong advocate of registration legislation.[7] Mrs Bedford Fenwick, who founded the British Nurses' Association (BNA), believed that women entering nursing should possess a certain level of education, that the training of nurses should be standardized, and that trained nurses should be licensed by the state.[8] She saw a standardized system of nurse training as a means of ensuring professional regulation and of providing a rational system of nursing practice.[9] She also saw state registration as a means of regulating entry to nursing, ensuring the recruitment of desirable women from a higher social class who could be trusted to give a scientifically based nursing service.[10]

In pursuing state registration, Bedford Fenwick was also attempting to break the monopoly that the voluntary hospitals exercised in recruiting and training nurses and, in this way, she was promoting the professional and economic independence of nurses.[11] For this reason, many of the voluntary hospitals were opposed to state registration. With any change to the status quo, the voluntary hospitals could lose their influence as the principal employer and supplier of nurses and they would be obliged to employ nurses on terms set by a state regulatory authority.[12] The Nightingale system of probationership training was providing the voluntary hospitals with a relatively cheap, disciplined and compliant worker, whose conditions of employment and methods of training they also controlled.[13] They effectively controlled the entire nursing labour force, including private nurses, and it was this constituency that Bedford Fenwick was particularly concerned for; she sought to reorganize the nurse's contractual relationship with the fee-paying client.[14] She also sought to prevent the exploitation of nurses by hospital administrators and doctors, and to establish nurses as the controllers of the nursing profession.[15]

Florence Nightingale and some prominent matrons, including Eva Lückes of the London Hospital, opposed state registration of nurses.[16] Nightingale opposed state registration on the grounds that nursing was as much about personal and moral qualities as it was about technical knowledge, and she believed that such qualities could not be tested in a state examination.[17] Seen as crucially important for good nursing, the moral qualities of the nurse would also be lost in the process of examination and certification.[18] Nightingale also opposed state control of nurses, holding the school matron to be 'primarily responsible for the conduct and efficiency of the Nurses'.[19] Many hospital matrons in England feared that state registration would bring new restrictions that would limit the field for recruitment to nursing, or it might result in smaller provincial hospitals failing to gain approval as training hospitals.[20] Some believed that the involvement of the State in nurse training would implicitly undervalue reputable hospital training and, in that way, would curtail their ability to procure funds and recruit nurses.[21] State registration might also make it difficult to dismiss a nurse, no matter how unsatisfactory her moral qualities.[22]

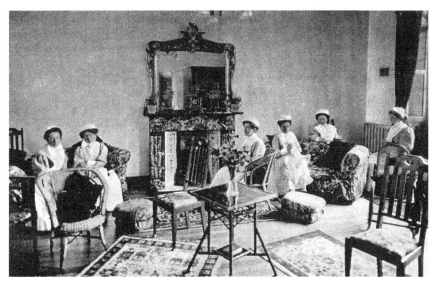

Figure 5.1 Nurses' sitting room, St Vincent's Hospital, Dublin, *c*.1910. Courtesy of the Irish Historical Picture Company

Select Committee on the Registration of Nurses

During the first two decades of the twentieth century, the campaign for state registration was the principal issue dominating nursing developments in Ireland and, in 1904, the Irish Nurses' Association (INA) and the Irish Matrons' Association (IMA) were founded to pursue the nursing cause and other professional interests.[23] With some four hundred nurses and matrons, fifty medical men and Mrs Bedford Fenwick in attendance, the INA held its inaugural meeting on 26 January 1904.[24] At the meeting, a resolution calling for the establishment of a Select Committee of the House of Commons to inquire into the nursing question was passed; the call was taken up by the vested interests in England, including the various nursing associations, medical men and MPs, and it resulted in the establishment of the Select Committee on the Registration of Nurses in June of 1904.[25]

Margaret Huxley, a founding member of both the INA and the IMA, was called to give oral evidence to the Select Committee, which sat during the years 1904 to 1905 'to consider the expediency of providing for the registration of nurses'.[26] Huxley's evidence typified the main arguments for state registration.[27] She pointed to the difficulties that individual nurses experienced in being ineligible to take up nursing positions outside of their own training hospital, and she gave evidence that many untrained nurses were passing themselves off as certified nurses. She also spoke of the poor quality of sick nursing in some nursing homes, which arose out of neglect and 'general frivolous behaviour' on the part of nurses. In Huxley's view, this behaviour resulted from a lack of supervision and a lack of proper training. She called for the establishment of a central regulatory authority for nursing, to 'lay down and define the term of training and what the education should be [and] … compel the hospitals to give a systematic training'. State examinations would ensure uniformity and would set the standard to be achieved. A standardized system of training under the control of a state regulatory authority would assure the public that nurses must be reputable women who 'know their work – the work they profess to know'. Huxley held that good nursing required intelligence and good clinical experience in training; the nurse in training should 'live the atmosphere of sickness'.

The Select Committee took evidence from thirty-four witnesses, including hospital matrons, superintendents of nursing institutions, practising nurses, representatives from the medical profession and from hospital management, civil servants and public representatives and, in its report, it supported the principle of state registration. Under state regulation, no person would be entitled to assume the title 'Registered Nurse' whose name was not on a register of nurses maintained by a central regulatory authority for nurses. The authority would admit to the register only 'such nurses as have had a training at a recognized training school for nurses', would determine what constituted a recognized training for nurses, and would have the power of inspection of training hospitals.

While the report of the Select Committee represented a victory for the pro-registrationists, state registration would not become a reality for a further fourteen years, during which time the Irish nursing associations and nursing leaders, principally Huxley, continued to lobby Parliament for registration legislation.[28] As a way of uniting the various pro-registration groups and associations in Ireland and England, a Central Committee for the State Registration of Nurses was established in 1909.[29] In this period, the Great War intervened. While the war delayed the processing of registration legislation through Parliament, it ultimately advanced the nursing cause, in that the contribution of nurses to the war effort greatly enhanced the public image of nurses and nursing. Margaret Huxley played her part in the war effort by coordinating the nursing services of the Dublin University College Hospital for Wounded Soldiers in Dublin Castle.[30]

The Irish Board of the College of Nursing and the Irish Nursing Board

In London in March 1916, with the support of many of the prominent voluntary hospitals in England, the College of Nursing was established. Its aims were to promote the advancement of nursing as a profession, the better education and training of nurses, the establishment of a register of certified nurses, and it would grant certificates and diplomas to nurses who successfully passed its prescribed examinations.[31] The governing body of the College of Nursing had a total membership of thirty-six, including six representatives from Ireland who met as the Dublin Committee of the College. In March 1917, an Irish Board of the College of Nursing replaced the Dublin Committee of the College. With a membership of twenty-two that comprised twelve nurses, medical men, and lay members, the Irish Board represented an attempt by Irish nurses to assert their independence of British nurses.[32] Its membership included eight matrons of prominent hospitals in

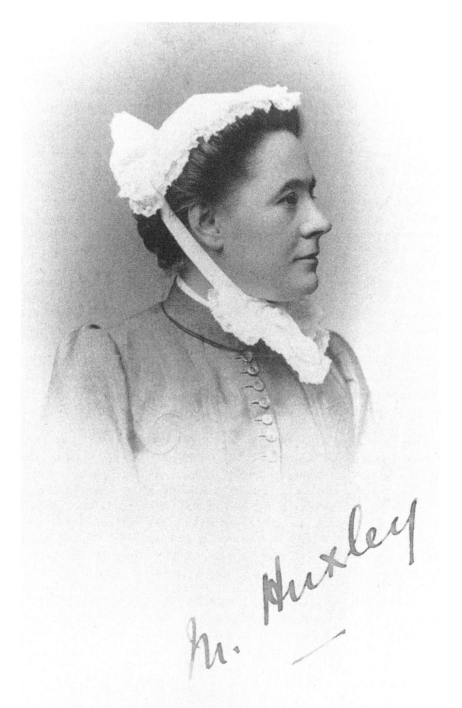

Figure 5.2 Margaret Rachel Huxley, Matron, Sir Patrick Dun's Hospital, Dublin.
Courtesy of the Faculty of Nursing & Midwifery, RCSI

Dublin, Belfast, Limerick and Waterford, and it included Miss Egan, President of the Irish Matron's Association.[33]

The Central Committee for State Registration of Nurses in London was opposed to the establishment of the College of Nursing, on the grounds that the College's scheme for voluntary registration would not achieve statutory registration. In Dublin, Margaret Huxley and the INA also opposed the establishment of the College of Nursing and the Irish Board of the College; they too believed that the pursuit of a voluntary system of registration did not go far enough in attaining regulation of the nursing profession. Huxley and the INA expressed their opposition to the Irish Board of the College of Nursing by establishing a separate and independent Irish Nursing Board in May 1917.[34]

The aims of the Irish Nursing Board were the formation of a register of all trained nurses, the improvement of nurse training, and the attainment of professional self-regulation by nurses; the Board's membership comprised four medical men, elected by the College of Surgeons, and twenty-two nurses, elected by nurses themselves.[35] The nurse members of the Board included Huxley and the matrons and lady superintendents of those Dublin hospitals not represented on the Irish Board of the College of Nursing.[36] The Irish Nursing Board conducted its business through quarterly meetings, and it received applications from nurses for registration. Every nurse could apply to have her name entered onto the register, having passed an examination set by the Board and having paid a fee. All registrants were entitled to vote in the election of the Board members and, in this way, nurses would 'manage their own affairs.'[37] Membership of the Irish Nursing Board would bring benefits not just to its members but also to the public, who could be guaranteed that the registrant had 'satisfied the Board as to her qualifications and training as a nurse'.[38]

Like the Central Committee on State Registration in England, the Irish Nursing Board rejected overtures from the College of Nursing to 'throw in their lot' with the College, arguing that the Irish Board of the College was not elected or in the control of nurses themselves and that it did not have statutory powers.[39] The Honorary Secretary of the Irish Nursing Board, Miss Carson Rae, expressed concern that the College proposed to issue two kinds of certificate, a certificate of proficiency and a certificate of training and proficiency, thereby 'mixing up trained nurses with other women workers in hospitals, to whom they also propose to grant certificates'.[40]

In the closing years of the campaign for state registration, there was concern that 'grave abuses' still persisted in relation to the position of the nurse. In 1917, Dr Thomas Percy Kirkpatrick, an active supporter of the Irish Nursing Board, noted that 'mere rank impostors' were posing as nurses to the detriment of the good name of the nurse, that nurse training schools had 'sprung up in all directions', and that some had given the rank and title of 'nurse' without having provided adequate instruction.[41]

Registration legislation and the first General Nursing Council for Ireland

Registration legislation for nurses was finally attained in 1919, but only after a series of bills had been brought before Parliament, the first of which was introduced in 1904.[42] For each successive year up to and including 1914, a nurses' registration bill went before Parliament but failed to get enacted.[43] In 1919, two bills proposing the registration of nurses were presented to Parliament. The Royal British Nurses' Association sponsored one bill while the College of Nursing sponsored the other. During the parliamentary debates, there was evidence of conflict between the two professional associations sponsoring their respective bills and, in the face of irreconcilable sectional interests, the Minister for Health Dr Addison introduced a new Nurses' Registration Bill on behalf of the Government.[44] The bill proposed the establishment of a General Nursing Council for England and Wales.[45] However, the Bill did not include provision for the registration of nurses in Ireland. So alarmed was the Irish pro-registration movement at this development that a deputation representing the INA, the IMA and the Irish Nursing Board travelled to Westminster and, after successful lobbying, secured the introduction of an Irish Nurses' Registration Bill.[46]

The Nurses' Registration (Ireland) Act of 1919 established the General Nursing Council for Ireland. The new Council was constituted with a membership of fifteen.[47] It was empowered to make rules for the purposes of forming, maintaining and publishing a Register of Nurses, regulating the admittance and removal of nurses from the Register, and regulating the conduct of examinations, which might be prescribed as a condition for entry to the Register.[48] The Council was also charged with making rules pertaining to the prescribed training and experience in nursing the sick, and rules pertaining to the approval of institutions for the training of nurses.

Comprising nine nurse representatives and five representatives of the medical profession, the General Nursing Council for Ireland held its first meeting on 25 February 1920.[49] The nurses members in attendance were Mrs Blunden, Miss Bostock, Miss Curtin, Miss Huxley, Miss Matheson, Miss Michie, Miss O'Flynn, Miss Reeves and Miss Walsh. The other members were Dr Edward Coey Bigger, Colonel Sir Arthur Chance, Mr R. J. Johnson, Dr P. T. O'Sullivan and Colonel William Taylor. The fifteenth member was the Countess of Kenmare, who was Vice-President of the Irish Branch of the Queen Victoria Jubilee Institute. Dr Edward Coey Bigger, who at the time was the Chairman of the Central Midwives Board, chaired the meeting and was unanimously elected as the first Chairman of the Council. At its second meeting, the Council elected Margaret Huxley as its Vice Chairman.[50] Members of both the Irish Nursing Board and the Irish Board of the College of Nursing were represented on the Council.[51]

At its first meeting, the Council quickly set about meeting its responsibilities under the 1919 Act. It appointed Major Geo. A. Harris as Registrar, on a salary of £300 per annum, and an assistant to the Registrar, on a salary of £100 per annum. The Council agreed to appoint nurses as permanent officers, 'when the

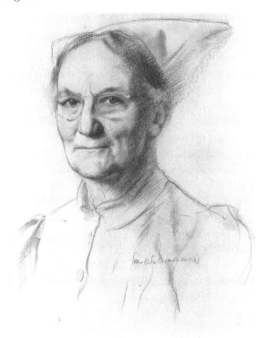

Figure 5.3 Alice Reeves, Matron, Dr Steevens' Hospital, Dublin. Courtesy of the Faculty of Nursing & Midwifery, RCSI

Council had settled down.' A Rules Committee was appointed to prepare the first set of rules relating to the conduct of the Council's business, the formation, maintenance and publication of the Nurses' Register, the admission and removal of nurses from the Register, and the conduct of examinations.[52] The conditions of admission to the Register required applicants to satisfy the Council that they had reached a sufficient standard of education, were of good moral character, and were not under twenty-one years of age.[53]

The Rules made provision for the admittance of existing nurses who had 'adequate knowledge and experience of nursing', and who had completed a period of at least one year of training in a recognized hospital. Provision was also made for the admittance of nurses who had commenced training prior to the promulgation of the Rules.[54] Grounds for removing a nurse from the Register included breach of the Rules, conviction of a felony, and a misdemeanour or other offence.

The Council Rules provided for the regulation of training and examinations and specified the required minimum duration of training as 'at least three years approved training and work in the medical and surgical wards of a hospital or hospitals.'[55] A list of subjects was prescribed; these were anatomy (six lectures), physiology (six lectures), hygiene (four lectures), bacteriology (two lectures), surgical nursing including gynaecology (nine lectures), medical nursing including fever and dietetics (nine lectures), and materia medica (five lectures). Candidates presenting for registration examinations were also required to have attained instruction in the theory of nursing that included attendance at thirty-six lectures of one hour each on the principles and practice of nursing to be delivered by the matron of the hospital at which the candidate was trained.

Examinations were prescribed in the various subjects. A Primary Examination, to be taken after eighteen months, would assess the probationer's knowledge of elementary anatomy and physiology, elementary materia medica, elementary bacteriology and hygiene, while a Final Examination would assess probationers in the principles and practice of medical, surgical, gynaecological and fever nursing, dietetics, nursing ethics, and invalid cookery. Examinations would be partly written, partly practical and oral, and candidates were permitted to take each part of the examination together or separately. The Final part could be taken only after the Primary part had been completed.

At its meeting of September 1920, the Council appointed a Registration Committee of eight persons, comprising the Council Chairman, five nurse members including Miss Huxley and Miss Reeves, and Sir William Taylor and Sir Arthur Chance. The matter of who among 'existing nurses' was eligible for registration quickly became a topic of the Council's deliberations. At the first meeting of the Council, Margaret Huxley had noted that the Irish Nursing Board already had four hundred trained nurses 'on their books' and she wondered if the new General Nursing Council would accept these nurses as 'existing nurses'.[56] Miss Matheson raised a similar concern in respect of nurses registered with the Irish Board of the College of Nursing. Fourteen nurses registered with the Irish Nursing Board were subsequently admitted to the Register on receipt of a payment of '£222 5% War Bonds plus a sum of £23. 3. 0' from the Board.[57]

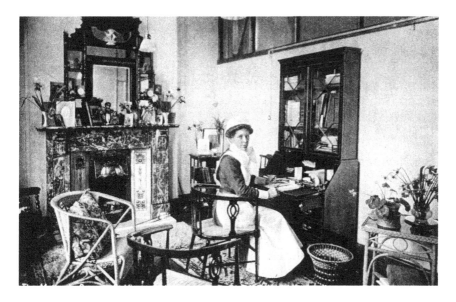

Figure 5.4 Miss Sutton, Matron, St Vincent's Hospital, Dublin. Courtesy of the Irish Historical Picture Company

The powers of the General Nursing Council for Ireland were questioned with regard to the Council's stipulation that one year of training was the minimum requirement for existing nurses to gain admittance to the Register. This matter was a particular concern, since it might exclude nurses already employed as 'qualified nurses' by the Local Government Board in the poor law infirmaries. The Rules Committee referred the matter to the Chief Secretary, who advised the Council that it did indeed have the power to 'impose a one year's training as a condition precedent to admission'.[58] The Rules also provided for the admittance of 'interim nurses' who had completed three years of approved training after the Nurses' Registration (Ireland) Act of 1919 was passed.

A special sub-committee of the Rules Committee was appointed to discuss with the Medico-Psychological Association the terms of admission to the Supplementary Part of the Register comprising Mental Nurses, but refrained from drafting any rules for the admission of male nurses, pending the action to be taken in England in that regard.[59] Having adopted the Rules, the Council resolved to forward copies of its Rules to the nursing councils in the United Kingdom, 'in order that an agreement on essential points might be obtained with these Councils'. The Council wished to ensure that its Rules should be 'in harmony with' the English Rules; following the advice it received from the various councils in the United Kingdom, the Rules Committee drafted a revised set of Rules pertaining to the admission of existing nurses. Conditions for the admission of male nurses and mental nurses were also included in the revised Rules, which the Council approved in June 1920. In an effort to ensure uniformity of registration procedures across the English, Scottish and Irish jurisdictions, a special conference was held in London in April 1921, and arising out of this conference, the English and Scottish Councils accepted the Rules of the Irish Council.[60]

The regulation of nursing through state registration was the single most important function of the first General Nursing Council for Ireland. At the end of 1921, a total of 220 nurses' names were entered on the General Part of the Register, while the supplementary parts for Mental Nurses and Infectious Diseases Nurses each contained the names of three nurses. The Council was empowered to refuse admittance to the Register, on the grounds that a nurse did not have the necessary approved hospital training. In October 1920, the Council issued a press notice intimating that nurses 'who desired to get on the Register should submit their application at once and in any event before 15th December 1921'.[61] The press notice generated a quick response from a large number of certified nurses and by March 1922 the Registration Committee reported that the total number of nurses on the Register was 920. Within two years, this number had risen to 3331, of which a majority of 2535 was entered onto the General Part of the Register.

Along with its function of maintaining a Register of Nurses, the regulation of nurse training was the other principal function of the first Council, and this latter function was expressed in three principal ways, namely the approval of hospitals as training hospitals, the preparation of a syllabus of training, and the establishment of state examinations. In 1923, the Council published a new syllabus and *Regulations for the Recognition of Hospitals as Training Schools for Nurses*.[62]

The regulations set out specific provisions in respect of hospitals training nurses for admission to the General Part of the Register, and separate provisions for hospitals training nurses for admission to the Supplementary Part.[63] A hospital seeking approval as a general training hospital was required to have a 'complete training school ... [with] at least one resident medical officer'. The hospital should satisfy the Council that it could furnish 'adequate training material and ... adequate staff and equipment for teaching, in accordance with the prescribed syllabus, for a three years' training'.

The regulations made provision for the amalgamation of two or more small hospitals, for the purpose of providing nurse training, and also permitted amalgamations of men's, women's, children's and 'special hospitals' for the same purpose. In 1923, a total of eleven hospitals in Dublin, three in Cork, and two in Waterford had received approval as training hospitals.[64] Candidates on the Supplementary Part of the Register could undertake general training on completion of two years of training in an approved hospital.

In establishing a system of state examinations, the Council appointed a Board of Examiners. The Board comprised qualified medical practitioners, who examined 'the theoretical part of the work', and registered nurses with not less than five years of experience and engaged in the teaching of nurses, who conducted the examinations in the practical part. Practical examinations required the attendance of three examiners, to include one Council member, one local examiner, and one examiner from Dublin or elsewhere. The pass standard was 50 per cent and a candidate was required to produce evidence of further instruction, in the event of her 'showing herself grossly ignorant of a subject or subjects'.

The deliberations of the first General Nursing Council for Ireland coincided with a time of momentous change in Ireland. When the Council was formed in 1920, the Irish War of Independence was ongoing and when hostilities ended with the Treaty of 1921, the Irish Free State of twenty-six counties was established and Northern Ireland was constituted as a separate jurisdiction of six counties. In Northern Ireland, a new and separate regulatory authority for nursing and midwifery, the Joint Nursing Council for Nursing and Midwifery for Northern Ireland, was constituted.[65] The General Nursing Council for Ireland was thereafter responsible for the regulation of nursing in the new Irish Free State. The first Council met on ninety-three occasions during its first term of office, and its tenure came to an end on 31 December 1923.

Issues and deliberations in the inter-war years

Within a few short years after the General Nursing Council for Ireland had assumed statutory responsibility for the regulation of nursing in Ireland, the Free State Government had assumed control of the various offices of state, and the London Government's branches of administration in Ireland had been dismantled and replaced by the government departments of the new State.[66] Responsibility for public health came with the portfolio of the Minister for Local Government and the Department of Local Government; the Department administered the health services through central and local government structures that included the county councils, the Board of Assistance and the Hospitals Commission.[67] Dáil Éireann, the Free State Government, replaced the poor law boards of guardians with the Board of Assistance, abolished the poor law unions, and set about rationalizing hospital services on a county and district basis.[68] In the process, a great many of the workhouse infirmaries became county hospitals and, by the mid-1920s, financed by local rates and administered by local boards of health and public assistance, as many as sixty-four workhouses had been converted into county homes, county hospitals, and district or fever hospitals.[69] Along with the county hospitals, the voluntary hospitals continued to be the principal provider of indoor medical relief.

In 1924, a new General Nursing Council for Ireland was elected by a postal ballot of the more than two thousand nurses on the Nurses' Register. The new Council contained few of the members of the original Council; Margaret Huxley was among those to lose a seat at the election. The new Council included just four of its original appointees, the Chairman Sir Edward Coey Bigger, Dr O'Sullivan and two nurse representatives, Margaret O'Flynn and Margaret Walsh.[70] Its new members were doctors Meenan, Blaney, Whittle, McBride and Harding, and nurses Herbert, Doyle, Smithson, Lanigan O'Keeffe, Phelan and Ellis. The Council met on 22 February 1924 and duly re-elected Sir Edward Coey Bigger as its Chairman.[71] Praising the achievements of the outgoing Council, the new Council resolved to 'live up to the high standard in everything affecting the good of the nursing profession which had been handed on to them by the members of the former Council'.[72] At its second meeting on 18 July 1924, the Council elected Mrs Annie Black RGN as the new Registrar and it appointed a new Rules Committee, which set about revising the first syllabus of training.

The first elected General Nursing Council for Ireland ended its term of office in 1929 and was replaced by a new Council. Sir Edward Coey Bigger was again re-elected as its Chairman, and the new Council agreed that it had the 'good fortune to have the benefit of Sir Edward's wise council and the guarantee of his strict impartiality'.[73] The 1929 Council was, in turn, replaced in February 1934 by a newly elected Council.[74] Throughout the inter-war period, the various councils debated a range of policy matters, including reciprocity with other national councils, the registration requirements for mental nurses, candidate selection, and council examinations.

In 1926, the Council discussed the 'growing practice of Boards of Health interfering with the Doctors and Matrons in the selection of Probationer Nurses'.[75] The Council was concerned that political interference and patronage could result in probationers being selected regardless of their fitness. If Boards could select 'none but their friends', there was the risk that unsuitable persons would gain entry to nursing. Aside from imposing a minimum educational standard for entry to nursing, the Council did not have a statutory function in the matter of candidate selection and, therefore, could not veto decisions regarding the selection of individual candidates. As the probationer's employer, the voluntary hospital maintained its independence from direct State control in its day-to-day administration, particularly in the areas of nurses' conditions of employment and the recruitment and selection of staff. Patronage remained a cause of concern for the Council in the inter-war years, but the matter was not rectified in the lifetime of the Council.[76]

Examinations were the subject of much debate in the Council. The Rules Committee agreed the Scheme for Conducting Council Examinations for state registration in 1925. The Preliminary Examination, to be taken at the end of the first year, and the Final Examination were held in January and June of each year. Physicians, surgeons and nurses conducted oral examinations, while the nursing members of the Council also conducted the practical part of the examinations. The written examinations were generally held in the principal urban centres, at such venues as University College Dublin, Bolton Street Technical Schools and University College Cork. The oral and practical examinations were conducted in the hospitals. Candidates failing the examination or any part thereof were required to re-enter for the entire examination.

Following the first round of examinations in 1925, the Council discussed the reported concerns of one examiner that nurses displayed great theoretical knowledge during the course of State oral examinations, but that 'they were not so good at the practical part of Nurses' training'.[77] In consequence of this concern, the Council wrote to all training schools drawing their attention to 'the need for an increased amount of instruction in practical nursing'. In 1927, the Council debated the separation of the medical and surgical parts of the practical examination. Dr Meenan proposed the separation, while Miss O'Flynn pointed out that the syllabus indicated how closely medicine and surgery were linked in the practice of nursing, and she urged that 'no compensation should be allowed when it was shown that a Nurse was very weak in Practical work'.[78] It was finally agreed that examinations should consist of three parts, namely written and oral examinations in medicine, written and oral examinations in surgery, and an examination in practical nursing. It was also agreed that candidates failing an examination were required to re-enter only that portion in which they were unsuccessful.

In 1931, on a recommendation proposed by Alice Reeves, Matron of Dr Steevens' Hospital, the Council considered the 'advisability of having a printed form for certificate of character for all candidates presenting themselves for the Council's Examinations'.[79] The Council rejected the proposal, on the grounds that it (the Council) would ultimately be responsible for turning down a nurse whose good character was not attested to. In the same year, the Council discussed the fact that the results in the Dublin examinations showed a higher failure rate than in the rest of the country.[80] Dr Meenan suggested that these variations were probably due to variation in the standard of examination across examination centres. Miss Halbert, Matron of St Vincent's Hospital, pointed out that, while acting as an examiner, she observed that 'in several cases, Candidates definitely failed by her had been passed as a result of the way very high marks were given by the other Examiner'. Arising out of Miss Halbert's observation, the Council discussed the advisability of appointing 'visitors' who could 'arrive without notice to see how the examination was being conducted'. A new scheme for conducting Council examinations, published in 1934, set out the variety and methods of examinations, the pass standard and the conduct of examinations.[81] Under the new scheme, the final oral examinations would be conducted by medical examiners, while nurse examiners would examine candidates jointly in the practical examination. A declaration by the hospital matron to the effect that the candidate had attended at least 75 per cent of the course of lectures and had received the required training in the wards of the hospital became a new requirement for entry to the final Council examinations.

Survey of hospitals

The *Regulations for the Recognition of Hospitals as Training Schools for Nurses*, published in 1931, contained the provision that affiliated groups of general and other hospitals, when adjudged to be sufficiently large when working together, could seek approval as a training school.[82] During the 1930s, the Council considered numerous applications from small regional hospitals for approval as affiliated training schools.[83] However, the Council refused several applications on the grounds that the institutions did not meet the Council's criteria for approval. Arising out of the many applications that it received, the Council's Hospitals Committee conducted a survey of all the recognized training hospitals in the Irish Free State, requesting them to 'state their facilities etc. for the purpose of nurse training'.[84] The aim of the survey was to 'examine the whole question of affiliated training schools recognized by the General Nursing Council in regard to equipment, accommodation, staff and facilities for training generally'. The survey elicited a poor response from the training hospitals, with just thirteen hospitals returning the completed questionnaire. Of this number, only two hospitals, the Bons Secour Hospital, Cork and the Mercy Hospital, Cork, were 'complete training schools', while the remainder were either 'affiliated' or 'amalgamated' training schools.[85] Dr MacCarville, a member of the Hospitals Committee who compiled the report of the survey, noted:

> In the majority of cases the questionnaire was inadequate; in many cases evasive and misleading; and with a few exceptions generally unsatisfactory. The great majority did not, as requested, supply details of the lectures and by whom given. Some who did showed that they were unaware of the course prescribed by the syllabus. One showed that the surgeon devoted eight hours weekly to lecturing the nurses, while in direct contrast another showed that the lectures were given entirely by sisters and none by a doctor. Four had no skeleton for anatomical lectures. One had no skeleton, no R.M.O., no model, no lay-figures, made no return of lectures given but charges a premium. One had six trained nurses, sixteen probationers, over 200 beds; an average bed occupancy of 153; i.e. one trained nurse per an average of 25.3 patients.[86]

The survey revealed that in a large number of the cases there was 'an absence of proper organization in the matter of training facilities in the hospitals at present recognized by the Council'. Dr MacCarville observed that, while all the hospitals had been previously recognized as training schools by the Council, it might be the case that some were 'not carrying out their trust to the Council in a bona-fide manner'. While some hospitals showed 'an excellent effort to afford adequate training', others were 'handicapped by an unfortunate alliance'. Dr MacCarville concluded that 'considering the advances in medicine, improved hospital equipment, and the training efficiency expected from an up-to-date general nurse', the only way of meeting the question of training was to draft an entirely new set of regulations. To this end, he recommended that a sub-committee should be appointed to prepare the new regulations, indicating the minimum general requirements of a hospital, the minimum equipment, the 'type of work' in which a hospital must be engaged, and the ratio of probationers to registered nurses.

On Dr MacCarville's recommendation, the new Rules Sub-committee duly prepared the revised regulations and presented them to the Council for approval in 1937. The revised regulations set down a number of specific conditions that a hospital seeking approval as a training school should meet. These included the requirement to have a bed occupancy of no less than fifty patients, with segregation of medical and surgical patients in separate wards, and have gynaecological and children's beds, outpatient, casualty and X-ray departments. The hospital should have one medical officer, one matron, one tutor sister and regular visiting staff, to include one physician, one surgeon, one gynaecologist and one radiologist. The regulations stipulated that 'lectures on the full course of subjects prescribed in the Council's Syllabus be given systematically and in regular series'.[87] The new regulations also imposed stringent conditions on those hospitals seeking approval as amalgamated or affiliated hospitals, including the stipulation that the Council could approve no hospital without prior inspection and subsequent regular inspections. Probationers in affiliated training schools would be required to complete their training in the complete training school to which their hospital was affiliated. The Rules Sub-committee later recommended that the system of affiliated or grouped hospitals be maintained only for the purpose of providing for preliminary training, and it recommended the abolition of the system on the grounds that it was undesirable.[88]

Having obtained ministerial approval in 1938, the Council's revised regulations were circulated to all hospitals providing nurse training. The system of amalgamated and affiliated training schools was clearly unsatisfactory in the eyes of the Council. Smaller hospitals that did not measure up to the criteria for approval, particularly in terms of their level of clinical activity and/or their resources for teaching, would not be permitted to continue to act as training schools. By imposing new stricter conditions under which they could operate in future, the Council was effectively acting to phase out or greatly curtail the affiliated training schools.

Conclusions

The campaign for registration legislation started quickly after the late nineteenth-century nursing and sanitary reforms, and the campaign was an extension of the same reform process. Vested interests, professional disunity and the Great War all contributed to a protracted campaign, and its conduct reflected divergent views on the function of professional regulation. Professional regulation through state registration represented the final act in the reform of nursing, and Irish nursing contributed in a significant and effective way to the achievement of registration legislation. As an act that put nursing on a professional footing, state registration was the single most important milestone in the development of modern nursing.

In the years leading up to state registration, the trained nurse in Ireland was viewed as 'one of the essentials of civilized life'.[89] This elevated social position of the nurse, the entry of influential women into key positions of leadership in nursing, the support of the medical profession, the improvements in care that nursing reform had brought, and the role that nurses played in the Great War all contributed to the ultimate success of the nursing cause. While not inevitable, the attainment of state registration was a predictable consequence of the confluence of developments that included progress in scientific medicine and women's suffrage.[90] Many advocates of state registration were also advocates of women's suffrage, and the movement for state registration paralleled the movement for women's franchise.[91]

In his seminal work, Brian Abel-Smith describes the campaign for state registration as 'a battle for status conducted against a background of rampant snobbery and rampant feminism'.[92] Hector argues that the supporters and opponents of state registration were motivated by mixed and obscure motives that included financial interests and concerns over power and authority.[93] Bradshaw points out that while both sides in the campaign agreed on the vocational ethos of nursing and while both upheld the integration of theoretical and practical instruction in the apprenticeship-training model, in essence, the dispute was about the relative importance of intellect/technical competence and moral character.[94] While the principal aim of the campaign was the regulation of nursing, a number of interrelated sub-plots were being played out in the course of the campaign, including women's emancipation, the control of employees, and the locus of power and authority over nurses.

The Nurses Registration (Ireland) Act of 1919 established the General Nursing Council for Ireland; the Council regulated nursing for the first thirty years following Irish independence. The first Council's tenure coincided with the abolition of the poor law system and a restructuring of medical relief in Ireland. The Council would be replaced in 1950 at a time when the notion of a welfare state was emerging in Britain and Ireland.[95] Therefore, both the establishment of the Council and its disestablishment were timely, in that both events coincided with important developments in Irish healthcare policy.

Aside from establishing the Register of Nurses, the most outward expression of professional regulation was the standardization of nurse training. However, while the General Nursing Council for Ireland now regulated the profession and while its rules and regulations determined much of the probationer's curricular experiences, the probationer's position as the principal provider of nursing service in the hospital wards did not change. Her curricular experiences were shaped by the stance of independence adopted by the voluntary hospitals in determining their own nursing policy in areas like recruitment and selection and the organization of the curriculum. This was the case before the attainment of state registration and it remained so after state registration. The voluntary hospital was a complex social world of hospital managers, doctors, matrons, lady superintendents and nurses, and the probationer's day-to-day curricular experiences were shaped as much by the events and activities of this complex micro social world as they were by the decisions of any national regulatory authority.

6 'Knowledge of her work'
The curriculum *c*.1899–1949

In the fifty-year period following the reform of hospital nursing, principles and patterns in the methods of organizing instruction were established and refined. Curriculum structures included the programme of systematic teaching and uniform examinations offered by the Dublin Metropolitan Technical School for Nurses and the preliminary training school system that emerged in the 1940s. Throughout the period in question, principles of curriculum and instruction were discernible in the content of instruction and examinations; following state registration in 1919, these principles gave rise to the various rules, regulations and syllabi that were published by the General Nursing Council for Ireland. Some of the ways that the hidden curriculum found expression provide evidence of the values that underpinned the curriculum.

Modus operandi

The curriculum was designed to prepare the probationer for her clinical role as a nurse. Her curricular experiences reflected the extant beliefs concerning the knowledge and skills needed for the performance of her clinical role and beliefs concerning the kind of a person that she ought to be. Her experiences were also aimed at socializing her into her profession and into the hospital system where she would most likely work when trained.

Practical experience in sick nursing supported by theoretical knowledge was seen as essential to learning the art of nursing. The practical and theoretical aspects of training were held to be interdependent, and the notions of the *art* and *science* of nursing were frequently used to illustrate this interdependence. In 1914, James Cantlie, surgeon and the author of the *British Red Cross Society Nursing Manual*, wrote:

> No man or woman can become an efficient hospital orderly or nurse merely by listening to a course of lectures or by reading a textbook on nursing. On the other hand, without instruction by lectures and reading, experience is but ill-founded and is calculated to develop a mere 'hospital hand' in contradistinction to an intelligent assistant to the physician or surgeon in dealing with disease ... those intending to nurse the sick must have the science of their calling taught them before they are qualified to practice [sic] the art.[1]

This view was the basic tenet upon which the curriculum was organized; theory would precede practical experience. While the nurse could gain a thorough understanding of her work in advance, this would be redundant without the benefit of experience in the practicum. Indeed, too much scientific knowledge could be attained at the expense of practical know-how, and it might also mask incompetence and ineptitude, as one writer of a nursing textbook observed in 1893:

> It may be … that there is a danger underlying the actual position of a trained Nurse, which we should do well to bear in mind – the risk, that is, of scientific knowledge covering up and putting out of sight the value of homely detail, and small matters connected with a patient's comfort and well-being.[2]

Nursing required a 'dextrous aptitude' that could only be developed through practical experience, and theoretical instruction was intended to supplement 'the more important practical training' that the nurse received in the hospital ward.[3] The pre-eminence of practical experience over scientific theory was the official orthodoxy in nurse training and this orthodoxy ensured that the probationer spent most of her training in the hospital ward. It also permitted nursing reformers to introduce and sustain the apprenticeship-training model.

In order to fulfil her role as a hospital nurse, it was held that the nurse needed to know something of the nature of disease, its signs and symptoms, its pathology and its treatments. This 'clinical knowledge' was necessary for rational observation of the sick. Through lectures, physicians and surgeons transmitted much of this clinical knowledge, and in the process provided probationers with a form of medical knowledge that they abridged and adapted to the needs of the nurse.

Instruction was provided through the medium of the lecture and through the written medium of the new nursing textbooks, which presupposed literacy.[4] Through the lecture, the doctor conveyed to the probationer the importance of her role in continuously observing and supervising the patient and she learned that the 'cultivation of the faculty of observation' was most important for a nurse.[5] As she observed signs, symptoms and responses to treatments, the nurse was expected to understand their significance. On this basis, she received instruction in anatomy and physiology, the action of drugs, and the meaning of signs and symptoms. Knowledge of elementary physiology was viewed as essential in the nursing of 'very intricate [and] constantly changing' medical cases.[6]

Instruction was also given in other aspects of sick nursing, including the management of fever cases, invalid cookery, and giving medicines.[7] In examinations, the probationer was expected to write about aspects of nursing theory, such as the signs of inflammation, the sources of contagion, the use of a surgical dressing and the nursing care of specific medical and surgical cases.[8] She was required to learn elements of theory in an integrated way; subjects like physiology and bacteriology were usually examined in conjunction with nursing subjects.

By the end of the nineteenth century, hospital medicine had evolved into a number of distinct sub-disciplines, including medicine, surgery, ophthalmology, aural medicine, gynaecology and orthopaedics, and specialist clinical departments were also set aside for accidents, sick children and the treatment of infectious diseases. The probationer worked in these various clinical departments where she was exposed to a wide variety of clinical cases so that she might develop a broad repertoire of nursing skills.

Clinical instruction prepared the probationer for her role as a worker in her training hospital or in private nursing. During clinical placements, teaching was an explicit pedagogical activity. At the Richmond Surgical Hospital, probationers were permitted, 'under sister's eye', to do some surgical dressings and take out stitches and they carried out a range of tasks included temperature taking, giving enemas, care of the mouth and pressure points, catheterization, application of poultices, rectal feeding and giving medicines.[9] Such tasks involved complex skills that could not be performed safely without prior instruction from the certified nurse. Aside from routine ward work, the probationer was expected to attend doctors' rounds and listen to the clinical lectures that were given to the medical students. While it involved ward-based instruction by the unit sister and by the lady superintendent, much learning in the practicum was incidental, occurring in and through the performance of clinical duties and tasks. Probationers at the Richmond Surgical Hospital were awarded marks for ward work, indicating that some assessment of their clinical performance took place.[10] A probationer could not go forward for examinations without having first attended the required clinical placements and, where she lacked the skills to nurse effectively, the lady superintendent had the power to prevent her from going forward for examination.

In the period before state registration, a number of educational principles were established that would remain the basis of instruction in the training of nurses. Working and learning under the supervision of the trained nurse was the essence of apprenticeship training and this method of instruction was the principal feature of the earliest nurse training schemes. As an instructional model, apprenticeship training gave exposure to a variety of clinical cases and expanded the probationer's repertoire of clinical knowledge and skills. The epistemological distinction between theoretical and practical instruction was also established in the period.

The medium and the message

Aside from the instruction given in lectures and demonstrations, the textbook was the other principal medium of instruction. In the early 1900s, a range of textbooks for nurses was available. These included textbooks written by nurses, such as *Notes on Nursing* by Florence Nightingale (1860), *Hints on Nursing* by Mena Drew (1889), and *Hospital Sisters and their Duties* (1886) and *Lectures on General Nursing* (1892), both written by Eva Lückes.[11] Doctors wrote many textbooks, including *Notes on Medical Nursing* (1897) by James Anderson and the *Red Cross Society Nursing Manual* (1914) by J. Cantlie.[12] Textbooks were also available on such topics as materia medica, dietetics, and anatomy and physiology.[13]

As a medium of instruction, the nursing textbook functioned as a technical manual that offered detailed step-by-step rules of procedure. It also functioned as a medium for transmitting messages, and in this way it was a pedagogical tool that mapped out authority relations in the workplace.[14] The textbook also transmitted nursing values, such as the value of hard work, hospital economy, truthfulness, and loyalty to the institution. It conveyed the relative value placed on aspects of nursing care, such as attentiveness to the patient's needs, alertness to sudden changes in the patient's condition, attention to detail, and accurate and honest reporting. Truthfulness was frequently stressed, since reliable and accurate reporting by the nurse was essential for the successful conduct of clinical medicine, where the physician or surgeon was in attendance for only a relatively small part of the patient's day.[15]

Textbooks written by medical men were an important medium for doctor–nurse communication; through the medium, the doctor communicated directly with each individual nurse, imparting medical knowledge and communicating his views on the nurse's role and status, her responsibilities to the doctor, and her place in the hospital structure.[16] In a pamphlet written by the Dublin physician Thomas Percy Kirkpatrick, entitled *Nursing Ethics* and published in 1917, the reader was reminded of her responsibilities as a nurse in training:

> One of the first duties of a nurse at the start of her training is to gain as thorough a knowledge as she can of her work. The more thorough that knowledge is the more efficient her services will be; and what a tragedy may wait on ignorance, especially if that ignorance be the result of one's own carelessness and neglect of opportunities …[17]

The reader was entreated to 'strive with all her might to be thoroughly efficient both in her studies and in her work'. While the pamphlet was ostensibly a treatise on nursing ethics, Dr Kirkpatrick took the broadest interpretation of that subject, wasting no opportunity to treat of the responsibilities of the nurse:

> Every nurse in hospital will be compelled to work hard; but every nurse should try to do that hard work thoroughly … What is worth doing is worth doing well; and anything that is not done as well as we can do is done badly … No part of the nurse's work is so difficult as the management of her hospital patients. Nothing shows her good qualities so quickly as success in this management … Attention to detail and thoroughness in the discharge of one's duties are of great importance in hospital work.[18]

The nurse had a social responsibility to obey the hospital rules and such obedience reflected loyalty to the hospital. As a trusted officer of her training hospital, she owed it 'a whole hearted and loyal service', and she was cautioned that she should do nothing that might damage the good name of her hospital. Mindful of the prevailing financial circumstances of the voluntary hospitals, Dr Kirkpatrick also reminded his reader of her duty of 'strict economy' in order to ensure that the funds of the hospital were not wasted.

The nurse should not transgress the clinical jurisdiction of the doctor, whom, it appears, was unlikely to make erroneous clinical decisions, and she should make no autonomous clinical decisions regarding prescribed treatments without the gravest deliberation on her part.[19] She was not permitted to act independently of the doctor and she should follow the doctor's instructions without deviation.[20] Dr Kirkpatrick stressed the nurse's responsibilities in monitoring and reporting on the patient's progress, and he was unequivocal in delineating the boundaries of the nurse's clinical jurisdiction:

> It is no part of the duty of the nurse to direct the treatment of the patient; she carries out that treatment under the direction of the medical man, and so long as she remains with the patient it is her duty loyally to fulfill this task. Circumstances may arise when it would be her duty to protest, but such circumstances are very rare. Any apparent exception to this general rule must be scrutinized with great care before she allows it to determine her actions.[21]

From the pages of her textbook, the nurse could have no doubt that her clinical jurisdiction had its derivation in the prerogative of the doctor. Statements on the nurse's responsibilities to the doctor were not confined to the pages of textbooks written by doctors; in Drew's *Hints on Nursing*, the reader was instructed in how to make ready the sick room for the visit of the medical man:

> Everything must be in order when the doctor pays his visit to the patient. There must be no fuss or confusion. All information as to the patient's symptoms must have been previously obtained by the nurse, so that the medical man may not be detained longer than needful … and the nurse must look clean, fresh and cheerful, ready to receive the doctor. If the case is an infectious one, fresh disinfectants must have been sprinkled about freely. It is not right that the physician should be exposed to more risk than needful in visiting a patient … The nurse must write down all the doctor's directions immediately after he leaves the sick room, so that she may not forget them.[22]

The textbook advised the nurse on what her demeanour should be in the sick room; since her own disposition could influence the sick person, she should be calm and unhurried in her work, with a 'cheerful temper' and a 'calm hushed presence'.[23] She was expected to show self-control and no outward signs of revulsion or discomfort, when faced with unpleasant sights or unpleasant tasks.[24] Through the textbook, the nurse was also reminded of her social position and she was advised that in home nursing she would frequently meet a class of people that 'may not be those with whom she would wish socially to associate'; in such instances, she should 'try in every way consistent with her duty, to accommodate herself to her surroundings.'[25]

The value of good personal health was also conveyed in the textbook, and the nurse was instructed on how she should maintain her own health:

> The nurse must keep her bowels regular by taking some simple saline … she must wash the whole of her body once a day in cold water. Once a week she

must wash all over in warm water with soap. Her teeth should be brushed morning and night. An hour's exercise once a day in the fresh air is absolutely necessary. Her diet must be nourishing and she must not have her meals in the sick room. If she feels the least out of order, she must speak to a doctor.[26]

In its function as a technical manual, the textbook reveals something of the nature of clinical nursing care that the nurse was likely to proffer, and it offers glimpses into the stage of the development of nursing science and practice in the period in which it was published. While written as an instructional manual for use by members of Red Cross Voluntary Aid Detachments (VADs) of the British Red Cross Society, *The British Red Cross Society Manual for Nurses* was also written as a manual for all nurses. Published in 1914, it contained chapters on 'details on nursing', 'feeding the patient', 'bathing', 'invalid diet' and 'medicines and their administration', and its pages were replete with detailed instructions on how to carry out a range of technical tasks, such as giving beef tea, taking the temperature and taking the pulse. On the latter task, the highly prescriptive style was typical of this and similar instructional manuals of the period:

> To take the Pulse. – (a) Stand or sit according to the position of the patient, on the outer side of the right or left upper limb. (b) Place three fingers, (the fore the middle and the ring) of the right hand on the radial artery, about half an inch from the outer (radial) or thumb side of the forearm, and with the central of the three fingers one inch above the front of the wrist; at the same time place the thumb of the hand with which the pulse is being felt behind the forearm so as to support it …[27]

The concise steps set out in the foregoing passage were accompanied by underlying principles of the procedure that included information on the qualities of pulse, such as normal frequency and rhythm, and intermittent and irregular pulse. A passage on how to take the temperature was accompanied by a treatise on the causes and clinical signs of subnormal and above normal body temperature, and details on the design of the mercury clinical thermometer.

Dublin Metropolitan Technical School for Nurses

In the late nineteenth century, the demand for a standardized system of nurse training was an integral part of the case for state registration and the successful introduction of such a system would greatly advance the cause of the pro-registrationists. In Dublin, Margaret Huxley and a number of like-minded hospital matrons and medical men set about introducing such a system when they established the Dublin Metropolitan Technical School for Nurses in January 1894. Founded as 'a place for the better technical education of nurses in Dublin', the School was constituted as a centralized training school for the principal voluntary hospitals in the city.[28]

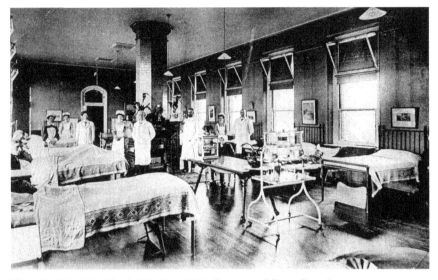

Figure 6.1 Ward 12, Meath Hospital, 1900. Courtesy of Peter Gatenby

The School provided systematic teaching and uniform examinations; at a cost of £1 per probationer, instruction consisted of three terms of three months each year. Each term comprised a schedule of twelve lectures in elementary anatomy and surgical anatomy in the first term, physiology and administration of drugs in the second term, and hygiene and invalid cookery in the third term. At the conclusion of each term, probationers took an examination in the various subjects and a list of the names of probationers from each participating hospital was prepared in order of merit and transmitted to their respective matrons. On passing the examinations, each probationer received a diploma from the Governing Authority of the School, certifying her knowledge in the subjects examined, and no probationer was permitted to receive a diploma without having first attained a hospital certificate indicating her proficiency in clinical nursing.

The School's Governing Authority comprised the matron and one representative of the medical staff of each of its affiliated institutions.[29] Margaret Huxley, then Lady Superintendent of Sir Patrick Dun's Hospital, was the School's first Honorary Secretary.[30] The School's affiliated institutions included the Nurses Training Institution at Usher's Quay, the Dublin House of Industry Hospitals, Dr Steevens' Hospital, Sir Patrick Dun's Hospital, and the Orthopaedic Hospital. Aside from the instruction received at the School's premises in Molesworth Street, probationers also attended demonstrations in invalid cookery given by Miss Bassett at the National Training School in Kildare Street.[31]

In its first twenty years, the School operated from a number of premises in Dublin, including the Molesworth Street premises, an office in Sackville Street, and No. 34 St Stephen's Green. The School was prominent in the training of nurses in Dublin in the years leading up to the enactment of the Nurses

Registration (Ireland) Act of 1919, and, at the time of state registration, the principal voluntary hospitals in Dublin were following the School's programme of systematic teaching and uniform examinations.[32]

Aspects of instruction under the General Nursing Council for Ireland

In regulating training schools and in introducing a national syllabus and examination system, the establishment of the General Nursing Council for Ireland in 1920 represented a significant milestone in the development of the nursing curriculum. However, since the membership of the Council was composed of hospital matrons and medical men, the curriculum continued to reflect the range of clinical activities occurring within the hospitals and related developments in clinical medicine. Since the probationer remained in the role of principal provider of the hospitals' nursing service following state registration, the content of instruction continued to reflect her learning needs for that role.

In the years after the establishment of the General Nursing Council for Ireland, the Dublin Metropolitan Technical School for Nurses continued to play a prominent part in the training of nurses in Dublin. The School provided the Council with a model for a standardized system of nurse training, and its programme of instruction was the standard to which other nurse training institutions subscribed.[33]

Some years after state registration, the School declared that all the clinical hospitals in Dublin, with the exception of the City of Dublin, the Mater

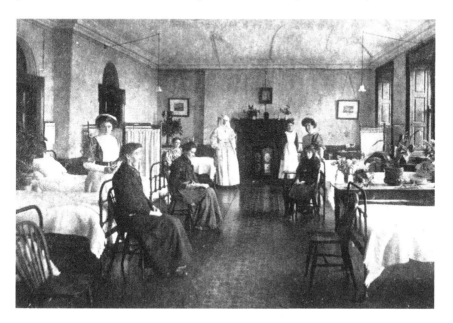

Figure 6.2 'The most important practical training …' St Anne's Ward, St Vincent's Hospital, Dublin. Courtesy of the Irish Historical Picture Company

Misericordiae, St Vincent's and the Charitable Infirmary, availed of the School's programme of lectures, and its Governing Authority reported there was great rivalry as to which hospital could obtain the medals for best marks.[34] During the 1930s and 1940s, the School's schedule of lectures was delivered at premises at No. 101 St. Stephen's Green, which the School acquired in 1926.[35] The School continued to function as a centralized training school for the hospitals of Dublin up until 1969, by which time individual hospitals had assumed responsibility for providing theoretical instruction.

The results of a survey of training hospitals conducted by the General Nursing Council for Ireland in 1936 highlighted the fact that many small hospitals appeared to be conducting nurse training with little reference to the statutory provisions set down by the Council.[36] Some smaller affiliated training schools were unaware of the course prescribed in the Council's syllabus and, in some instances, there were deficiencies in the resources for teaching and in the level of clinical activity necessary to support nurse training. While the large voluntary hospitals did not participate in the Council's survey, and while they had a propensity to guard their independence and to resist State interference in their affairs, they could not, in principle, develop and operate individual curricula without reference to the Council's regulations and syllabi. All of the hospitals were obliged to prepare their probationers for the Council's biannual examinations. Since the examinations represented the foremost expression of the Council's regulatory function in the curriculum, the Council had an indirect presence in the hospital training schools. The names of successful candidates were published in the professional press and this fact meant that the voluntary hospitals were keen to ensure that their probationers were well prepared for the State examinations. Institutional pride and, in some instances, institutional rivalry ensured that the hospitals expended much effort in preparing their probationers for the examinations. Moreover, the hospitals had a pragmatic interest in ensuring that their probationers were well prepared for examinations, since the content of the examinations reflected hospital clinical activity, and the probationer who was well prepared for examinations was also well prepared for her duties in sick nursing.

The needs of the voluntary hospitals were determining both the content of instruction and the content of the State examinations and, as hospital medicine developed and expanded, the nursing curriculum developed and expanded accordingly. Where individual hospitals offered specialist clinical services, curricula tended to reflect this; some hospitals provided additional instruction in such topics as neurology and urology. While subjects such as anatomy and physiology, materia medica, and pathology were included in the curriculum because they were seen as being necessary for the nurse's clinical role, their inclusion could convey to the public something of the status of the nurse. The public could see that since she studied the same subjects as the learned medical man, the nurse was both educated and intelligent; the Chairman of the General Nursing Council for Ireland, Sir Edward Coey Bigger, admitted as much when he wrote in 1937:

It may strike some that the inclusion of subjects [in the curriculum] which are not absolutely practical may be unnecessary, but the estimation of the importance of the profession by the public is to some extent guided by the standard of knowledge of kindred science displayed by individual nurses. It is partly in this way that the memory of the past, when the nurse was practically an untrained, ignorant and frequently intemperate woman of the type of Sarah Gamp, was swept away. A nurse must be a refined and educated woman who is acquainted with those sciences in which medicine is based as well as those practical points of nursing on which much of the comfort of the patients depend.[37]

With the advent of State examinations, the curriculum tended to be assessment driven, and evidence of this lay in the fact that a number of publications were produced with the aim of assisting nurses to prepare for the State examinations. For example, the Richmond Whitworth and Hardwicke Hospitals published *Practical Lectures According to the Syllabus of General Nursing Council for Preliminary Examination* in 1930.[38] The publication provides a window on the curriculum in the period. *Practical Lectures* contained lecture notes on a variety of topics, including 'hygiene of the patient', 'care of the back and prevention of pressure sores', and 'observation of excreta'. Lecture notes on aspects of the nurse's role in medical and surgical nursing were also included under such topic headings as 'administration of medicines', 'surgical technique, sterilization, etc.', and 'care of the patient before and after operation'. The inclusion of notes on dusting, cleaning, the care of bedding and disinfection of utensils implied that these activities were a part of the probationer's duties.

Practical Lectures also contained notes on maintaining the nurse's own health; this included advice on cleanliness of the body, avoiding fatigue and chilblains, and avoiding constipation, which it declared to be 'the root of most ill-health'. Like earlier nursing textbooks, the publication contained clear messages about the nurse's place in the hospital structure. It contained passages on 'the relation of a nurse to a doctor etc.', in which the reader was reminded that in the hospital 'the Surgeon or Physician is the superior', and that 'without being in any way familiar be as courteous as possible to a Doctor when he comes into the ward'. The probationer was not permitted to establish any untoward relationships with the patient:

> Never allow a patient to become familiar, once they do, the respect, which they should have disappears. The more aloof you keep, the better they will think of you.[39]

The textbook continued to be the medium through which values could be articulated and transmitted, and the reader of *Practical Lectures* was reminded of the values of obedience, truthfulness, punctuality and loyalty to the institution:

> Every nurse should be as loyal to her own training school as she should be to her own home ... she must add to its laurels, by not doing anything which would lose the least of its traditions.[40]

Many textbooks were written in a stylist idiom that made frequent use of the second person singular. In this way, the writer communicated directly with the reader. The tone adopted in most textbooks for nurses was one of *gravitas*, such that the reader was left in no doubt as to what was proper and improper in the nurse's professional and personal conduct.

Textbooks on a range of subjects allied to nursing became available after state registration, reflecting the incremental addition of new subjects. In 1941, the first edition of W. Gordon Sears' *Anatomy and Physiology for Nurses and Students of Human Biology* was published and was used by nurse training schools in Dublin.[41] New textbooks were also available in such diverse subjects as pharmacology, infection control, and psychology.

The content of examinations reflects the content of instruction and, in so doing, offers another window on the curriculum. Examinations also convey which aspects of instruction are implicitly valued in the curriculum and reveal the interdependent relationship between hospital medicine and nursing. The Preliminary Examination for 1931 contained the following items:

1   Describe the parts played in digestion by (a) the mouth (b) the liver.
2   How many milk teeth and how many permanent teeth are there? What are the functions of the teeth?
3   Describe the shoulder joint.
4   Write a note on the functions of the kidneys and the skin.
5   What are the boundaries, and name the contents of the thorax.
6   How would you treat severe haemorrhage from a ruptured varicose vein in the leg?[42]

In the corresponding examination in December 1939, candidates were required to answer questions related to the contents of the pelvis, the alimentary tract, the composition and functions of blood, and the functions of the skin.[43]

In the 1930s, hospital physicians and surgeons prepared the General Nursing Council's Final Examination papers. Candidates going forward for the Final State examinations were required to demonstrate knowledge of internal medicine and be conversant in specific terminology related to medicine and surgery, the pathological basis of signs and symptoms, and medical therapeutics, including pharmacology. The Council's Final Examination in Medicine in 1931 contained questions on topics related to bacteriology, dietetics, medical nursing, and materia medica and therapeutics, while the corresponding examination in 1939 contained questions on nursing in medical cases, including acute lobar pneumonia, acute nephritis, diabetes mellitus, duodenal ulcer, tuberculosis and typhoid, and drug overdose.[44] The examination paper in surgery in the same year included questions on fractured neck of femur, the treatment of a severe burn, the preparation and post operative care of total hysterectomy, and the signs, symptoms and complications of gall stones.[45]

The preliminary training school

In the 1940s, the nurse was expected to demonstrate 'considerable knowledge' of a wide range of subjects, including bacteriology, dietetics, materia medica, medicine, surgery and gynaecology.[46] The means of acquiring this knowledge was through a system of instruction organized around the probationer's work schedule; lectures were usually given in the morning or in the evening and preceding or following a duty shift. This system could not always guarantee that planned instruction would take place, since it was vulnerable to the vagaries of the clinical situation in the hospital. The probationer or, more likely, the lecturer might have to forgo a planned lecture due to an extended clinical workload.

By the mid-1940s, the ad hoc method of organizing instruction around the probationer's work schedule was being gradually replaced with a system that involved protected periods for instruction, and a number of hospitals in Dublin were giving planned instruction in the first weeks of training and before probationers took up their ward duties.[47] This arrangement was referred to as the 'preliminary training school', denoting the fact that instruction was aimed at preparing probationers for the General Nursing Council's Preliminary Examination at the end of the first year.[48] While the new system protected instruction in the first year of training, the practice of giving morning and evening lectures continued in the second and third years, and remained a feature of the training experience in some institutions up until the 1960s.[49] At about the time that the first preliminary training schools were introduced, the term 'student nurse' came into common usage.

The preliminary training school system gave scope for additional teaching and for planned study time. Sir Patrick Dun's Hospital introduced the system in 1944, when nine students were enrolled.[50] The preliminary training school premises were located at numbers 101 and 102 Lower Mount Street, where facilities included nine single bedrooms for student nurses, a fully equipped kitchen, dining room and bathroom, and accommodation for the Sister Tutor, comprising a bedroom, a sitting room and an office. The school's first Sister Tutor was Miss Anne Young, who went on to become Matron of the Charitable Infirmary and later founded the School of Nursing at St Kevin's Hospital. The Lady Superintendent Miss Chambers described the new system at Sir Patrick Dun's:

> Candidates enter the Training School for a period of twelve months. During this time they receive a full course of lectures as prescribed by the G.N.C. for the Preliminary State Examination. After three weeks in the School the students go to the wards three days a week from 2 until 4 pm. and help with the general ward work. One day a week a visit to some place of interest is made or a talk given by someone in charge of a special department – e.g., the Lady Almoner. Visits are paid to a Maternity Hospital, Orthopaedic Hospital, Industrial School, Child Welfare Centre, and Waterworks. When travelling facilities are available, we hope to take the students to farms where they may see the care and management of milk. On completion of Preliminary

Training, candidates are examined on all subjects taught in the Training School. If successful and suitable, they are then accepted for further training.[51]

The students also attended the wards for the routine work of 'sorting linen' on one morning per week. A 'test paper' was administered at the end of each week and following completion of each course of lectures, written and practical examinations were conducted in nursing, bandaging and sickroom cookery. Miss Chambers observed that while it was too early to form an opinion on the usefulness of the school, she expressed the belief that its introduction would be a great help to the ward sisters, nurses and patients:

> The preliminary training school should prove useful all round ... Knowledge of their practical work gained in the classroom should make them more efficient in the Wards from the start. Their patients and their Ward Sisters should benefit from this.[52]

Training in 'matters domestic' was included and this was integrated into the students' duties in the nurses' home:

> The nurses cook and serve their own meals in the Home. They are responsible for sweeping and dusting their own rooms, kitchen, bathrooms and lecture rooms. This was considered advisable in order to give them the requisite training in domestic affairs.[53]

While they were expected to attend to domestic matters, the student nurses at the first preliminary training school at Sir Patrick Dun's Hospital occupied a position of privilege over the students who entered training before 1944. The first group of nine 'PTS students' had separate quarters in the nurses' home and were prohibited from mixing with the other students.

In her annual report of 1945, Miss Chambers noted that the preliminary training school had 'proved a great success', and she observed that the high percentage of marks obtained in the recent State examinations gave great confidence.[54] While the preliminary training school system brought an improved training structure, the trainee continued to play a prominent role in the delivery of the nursing care in the hospital wards. However, the new system relieved the student nurse of the responsibilities associated with taking on the role of hospital nurse at the very start of her training, and when she did assume clinical responsibilities, she was better prepared.

Work, recreation and conditions of employment

With state registration and professional regulation, the probationer in the voluntary hospital might reasonably expect that her relatively high social status as a lady nurse would be further enhanced and that her economic position would improve with her new-found professional status. The probationer who harboured such expectations would be greatly disappointed. Her conditions of employment did not change following state registration and her economic position reflected the condition of relative poverty in which the new Irish Free State found itself during the period 1920 to 1950.[55]

The highly regulated regime of work and recreation, evident at the end of the nineteenth century, continued to be the probationer's abiding curricular experience in the decades following state registration. At the Royal City of Dublin Hospital in the 1920s, strict rules governed the probationer's work and recreation:

> [The Nurses and Probationers] are required to be quiet and orderly in their wards, passages, corridors and Nurses' Home. They must be strictly punctual in going on and coming off duty, and in their attendance at meals, lectures and classes ... [They] must keep themselves and the apartments allotted to their use neat and clean, making their own beds thoroughly before coming down to breakfast. They must at all times be ready to do such needle or other work as the Matron may direct.[56]

A student nurse's 'typical day' in the preliminary training school at Sir Patrick Dun's Hospital in the 1940s consisted of the following schedule of activities:

> 7.40 am Breakfast.
> 8.0 am On duty-Domestic duties.
> 8.30 am Lecture.
> 9.30 am Make bed. Tidy room.
> 10.0 am Study.
> 10.30 am Lunch.
> 11.0 am Lecture.
> 12.0 midday Study.
> 12.45 pm Prepare for Dinner.
> 1.0 pm Dinner.
> 2.0 pm Lecture.
> 3.0 pm Study.
> 4.0 pm Tea.
> 4.30 pm Study.
> 6.0 pm Off duty.[57]

Discipline was seen as a necessary part of the training of the nurse. In 1944, the *Irish Nurses' Magazine* carried an article entitled 'Hospital Discipline', in which the reader was entreated to see that her level of self-discipline was a measure of her suitability to become a nurse:

> It has to be recognized that submission to close supervision over a few years of training is a test not only of her moral stability but of her temperamental and even of her intellectual fitness for the career of a Nurse ... what she must bear in mind is that she will not always be a probationer any more than

she will always be a young girl, and meanwhile this graduation is as necessary for the career she ambitions as matriculation for entering a University or taking a certain Degree therein for the pursuit of a profession. In a word she is ascertaining, and the officials placed over her are assisting her to ascertain, whether or no she is merely a misfit and had better take some other profession.[58]

The reader was cautioned to avoid any behaviour that would be at variance with the expected conduct of a nurse:

nothing is more unbecoming in a young lady aiming at the dignity and responsibility of becoming a hospital nurse than hoydenish levity or thoughtlessness and reckless frivolity in the pursuit of some flitting entertainment out of place … that ought to be left to those giddy-headed young women who are fast making our era a byeword in history. The hospital nurse should be the model of decorum …[59]

While the demand for discipline and decorum conveyed hidden messages concerning the things that were valued in nursing, the probationer's conditions of employment also conveyed a message that the work that nurses performed had a relatively low value in the economic system. By the 1930s, over eleven hundred nurses were in training, the majority in the general voluntary hospitals. The ratio of trainees to qualified nurses was approximately 2:1, and nurses in training represented approximately one-fifth of the total national nursing workforce.[60] The nurse in training continued to represent an important material asset for the hospital, and this fact dictated many of her curricular experiences.

The probationer's situation became the subject of concern to nursing leaders and to some members of the medical profession. Speaking at a meeting called to discuss nurses' conditions of employment in 1942, Mr J. J. Fitzsimons, surgeon at the Richmond Hospital, asked rhetorically: 'One might well ask why does one become a nurse?' Mr Fitzsimons went on to depict the experiences of the probationer:

[She] enters hospital as a probationer, [and] during this trying time her vocation is tested to the full, with all the indignities, without any real nursing. From the start she has to struggle with lectures in anatomy, physiology, etc., these subjects have to be studied during her hours off duty, which are few and far between. She must submit to stricter discipline than a girls' school. Small breaches of discipline may cost her evening off … If during her probation she is found to be disobedient, frivolous, or to show signs of physical weakness, she may be sent home, and even after her probation period, if she fails to pass her examination within reasonable time she may be asked to resign. She must be in at 10 pm on her evening off, and if she wishes to go to a theatre or dance, she must ask for special leave. If there are any unfavourable reports from her sister, this leave may be refused.[61]

The speaker also observed that, due to the poor salary and difficult working conditions, the nurse had little to look forward to when her training was completed.
In addition, her clinical role left her at risk of contracting work-related infectious
diseases, such as tuberculosis, gastro-enteritis and diphtheria.[62] Tuberculosis was a
particular problem in the period and a survey of the health status of student
nurses at St Laurence's Hospital in Dublin for the period 1946–1950 indicated
that the disease was an occupational risk, with a number of deaths occurring
among the student population.[63]

Addressing a meeting of the Biological Association of Trinity College on the
problems of nurses in February 1944, Max Millard, a medical student from
Trinity College Dublin, commented on student nurses' working conditions.[64] He
remarked that the health of the nurse was neglected, that the nurse was 'bullied
(bullied in a manner that no one could now try on with maids), overworked and
underfed', and he described aspects of the working conditions of the student
nurse in the Dublin voluntary hospitals:

> For her health's sake, she is sent to bed early, and not allowed dances too
> often. Yet a common form of punishment is to refuse her off-duty so that she
> has to work fourteen hours. This must be very ennobling to her mind. It is
> also criminal. Moreover, for one reason or another, no Hospital has enough
> nurses. The result is that there are no reserves and if a nurse is off sick the
> hospital nearly caves in. Following from this is the fact that a sister is reluctant
> to let a nurse report sick to Matron unless she is obviously very ill. The Nurse,
> knowing the trouble it will cause, generally tries to appear well until she can
> bear it no longer. She considers too that sick leave is liable to be subtracted
> from her annual holiday and that a day in bed with a cold means her off duty
> for the month is gone.[65]

The speaker remarked that the attitudes of some of the student's superiors in the
hospital setting added to her difficulties:

> Who is more needful of a course in Group and Industrial Psychology than
> the sisters and matrons? So much ill-feeling is bred by misunderstanding and
> mishandling of difficulties, a lack of balance, a forgetfulness of the feelings of
> youth of 18–22 … Nurses look upon Matron as an autocrat to be feared, to
> whom the only thing to be said is 'yes Matron, no Matron'. The sister is only
> a smaller version of Matron. It leads to abuse of privileges and slackness as a
> show of discontent so that the Bosses have to exact some punishment to indi-
> cate that they are not to be slighted. To me this is one of the saddest aspects
> of nursing, for by it the nurse loses her chance of a more mature guide and
> adviser and seems to gain a little more unhappiness … no one in the world
> has a worse feeling of inferiority than the Nurse.[66]

Millard pleaded for 'a better psychological understanding of nurses by Matrons'.[67]
He also observed that many students did not receive formal instruction at the

commencement of training, declaring that the student nurse 'walks on at 7 am the first day and is walked on for the next month'.[68] Admonishing nurses for not standing by each other, he called on them to 'shake free of their lassitude', and he also called on his colleagues in the medical profession to support nurses and not to exploit them.

Addressing a meeting of the Irish Matrons' Association in October 1948, the Minister for Health Dr Noël Browne called for a more intelligent approach to the training and handling of nurses, observing that 'the modern girl requires more freedom than her predecessors, and allowance should be made for this'.[69] Dr Browne linked the shortage of nurses that obtained in the period to nurses' conditions of employment and to the perceived unattractiveness of the profession. In the following year, another Dáil Deputy remarked that probationers were treated 'more like a flock of sheep than anything else…they are afraid to complain'.[70] Nurses' working conditions were mentioned in a Dáil debate concerning the Estimates for Public Services in July 1948. One contributor Deputy Dr Brennan said that, in his capacity as a hospital administrator, he had witnessed the deleterious effects of poor living conditions on the health of nurses and, commenting on the regime of nurse training, he remarked:

> Its influence on a growing girl, between 19 and 21, is bound to have some effect on her nervous system, some effect on her outlook in life.[71]

Much of the commentary on nurses' conditions of employment emanated from members of the medical profession, who were to the fore in speaking on behalf of nurses. While nursing had its own independent voice, it appears that the corps of nurses was less inclined to speak out on matters of concern to nurses, either through apathy or through a sense of insecurity in employment.[72] The position of the nurse in training was especially insecure, since any outward expression of discontent could lead to serious sanctions, including termination of training. The procurement of employment, no matter how unpalatable were the pay and conditions, was important at a time of national economic hardship.

Conclusions

The needs of medicine and nursing in the voluntary hospitals and the rules, regulations and syllabi of the General Nursing Council for Ireland determined the content of instruction in the nursing curriculum. The values held by the nursing profession also gave rise to much that the probationer experienced in the curriculum. The curriculum functioned principally and explicitly to prepare the nurse for the performance of her working role. At the turn of the twentieth century, the nurse was trained for two principal roles, those of hospital nurse and private nurse. By the 1940s, her role as hospital nurse became pre-eminent and this role represented the principal justification for the curriculum.

Aside from its function of preparing the probationer for the work of sick nursing, the curriculum also functioned to socialize her into her chosen profession and into the hospital system. This latter function was achieved through the explicit messages contained in the content of instruction and through the implicit messages that were conveyed in the probationer's wider curricular experiences.

While the official curriculum declared that the nurse was being trained for a noble vocation and a responsible professional role in the health services, the hidden curriculum had less noble purposes, appearing to function to secure the nurse's submission to authority. The probationer was expected to accept discipline as a necessary part of her professional training, submit to a regime of close surveillance and behave in a decorous manner, and she was expected to be a loyal and efficient worker in the service of her training hospital. As a worker, she was required to work at maximum efficiency, to maintain her health and to develop the knowledge of her work. While the probationer experienced considerable economic hardship and a training regime that demanded subordination and docility, the voluntary hospitals continued to easily recruit young women into nursing.

In the period between the introduction of apprenticeship training in the 1880s and 1949, the last year of office of the General Nursing Council for Ireland, the curriculum underwent a process of gradual and incremental expansion to take account of new developments in scientific medicine and in related hospital nursing. Change also occurred in the way that the curriculum gradually moved from being an incidental and informal system of instruction towards a more structured programme, best exemplified in the preliminary training school system.

7 The Nursing Board and the training experience, 1950–1979

The establishment of a new Department of Health in 1947 indicated the growing importance of a publicly administered health service to the economic growth of the country and to the welfare of its people. Government health policy emerging in the post-war years emphasized public health and disease prevention and it aimed to expand health service provision and to improve access to the services. In this connection, policy on nursing envisioned a more rational approach to the recruitment and training of nurses, to take account of the national needs for a nursing service. Given the anticipated expansion of the nurse's role in the health services, policy was also concerned with the training of nurses and, in particular, with the requirement for nurses to study a broader range of subjects.

Health policy and nursing

The late 1940s was a transitional period in the development of health policy in Ireland, with efforts by the State to move from an overreliance on philanthropically based healthcare provision to state-funded provision.[1] Some of the impetus for this change came from the Beveridge Report, which was published in the United Kingdom in 1942 and which proposed a universal, publicly funded health service. Under the Fianna Fáil Government of 1932–1948, state-funded services were expanded through a hospital building programme, and the Government also set in place ambitious plans to provide a comprehensive national health service, free of charge to large numbers of the population.[2] These plans proposed free family doctor services, special services for mothers and children, and services for the prevention of infectious diseases.[3] When a new Department of Health was established in 1947, the functions of health and local government were separated, indicating that healthcare was an important and distinct element of Government social policy.[4] The Government's plans for the health services were interrupted with the defeat of Eamon de Valera's Fianna Fáil Government in the election of 1948 and its replacement by the first Inter-part Government, a coalition of five political parties under the leadership of John A. Costelloe of the Fine Gael Party.[5]

The period following 1948 saw much activity in the development of the health services under Dr Noël Browne, the Inter-party Government Minister for Health. Hospital services were made more accessible to a greater proportion of the population and a number of public health initiatives were successfully under-taken, including a TB eradication scheme and a programme of immunization. Dr Browne's programme of public health included plans for a free mother-and-child service, to be funded through a capitation payment. The scheme would be provided through a variety of services, including maternity and local authority hospitals, dis-trict medical officers, domiciliary health services, and through private general practitioners willing to participate in the scheme.[6] Like his predecessor, Dr Browne was attempting to introduce a de facto free national health service. However, the proposed scheme failed in 1951 due to a number of factors, including a lack of political support from all the members of his Government and strong opposition to 'state controlled medicine' from the hierarchy of the Roman Catholic Church and the medical profession.[7] Opposition was based on the view that state control of health services would transgress the rights of individuals and the family, and the scheme was seen to threaten the autonomy of the medical profession.

The Roman Catholic hierarchy and the medical profession continued to oppose the principle of State administered healthcare, notably the provisions of the Health Act of 1953, which included ambitious plans to extend the health ser-vices to greater numbers of the population. The hierarchy feared 'Government patronage with great risk of corruption,' while the medical profession feared 'complete control by the State of the medical profession'.[8] In meeting its responsi-bility to provide a universal health service to the population, the State was confronted by powerful vested interests in Irish social and political life that resulted in modifications to the plans of successive administrations during the 1950s. Despite this, the State succeeded in establishing a publicly controlled health service by the end of the 1950s. Although partly reliant upon the involve-ment of the relatively independent voluntary sector, the quality and range of services available and the level of access to these services had greatly improved. Public health services were being provided on the basis of a partnership between the State and the voluntary sector.[9]

Following the establishment of the Department of Health in 1947, efforts by the State to expand the health services would inevitably include consideration of nursing and midwifery services. The State's public health programmes, which included the hospital building programme and the various community health ini-tiatives, would necessitate a rational and coordinated approach to the regulation and training of nurses and midwives. With separate regulatory authorities, nurs-ing and midwifery were essentially separate and distinct disciplines. While the General Nursing Council for Ireland and the Central Midwives Board had served their respective professions well, there was the view in government that the time had come to put in place new structures for the regulation of nursing and mid-wifery.[10] The Minister for Health Dr Noël Browne first hinted at these new structures in 1948, when he had the Nurses Registration (Ireland) Act of 1919 under review.[11] Dr Browne was contemplating the establishment of a new statu-tory body to control the recruitment, training and employment of nurses. He held the view that 'the value of any health service depends largely on the efficiency of its personnel', and he believed that the health services of the future depended upon good education for a high standard of knowledge and skill.[12] He foresaw the establishment of a new national nursing board that would absorb the functions of both the General Nursing Council for Ireland and the Central Midwives Board. In the Minister's view, this change would 'facilitate the integration of the different branches of the nursing profession and the provision of the steady flow of nurses and midwives that will be needed for many years'.[13]

The publication of the Nurses Bill in 1949 confirmed the Minister's proposal to establish a new combined regulatory authority for nursing and midwifery.[14] This new authority would take on the existing functions of the General Nursing Council for Ireland and those of the Central Midwives Board, and it would be empowered to 'prescribe the manner in which and the conditions under which training shall be provided'.[15] During the second reading of the Nurses Bill in the Irish Senate in July 1949, Dr Browne spoke of the need to have an adequate supply of nurses in the health services, and he argued that the responsibility for ensuring this rested with the bodies responsible for regulating nursing and midwifery.[16] He concluded that the powers of the existing regulatory bodies were limited and that it was now necessary to 'approach the matter from the most effective manner in which the profession of nurses should be organized in the future'. Dr Browne considered that the powers of the proposed new regulatory body were vital to ensure the provision of properly trained personnel in adequate numbers for the nursing services in the years ahead.[17]

Dr James Deeny, the Chief Medical Adviser in the Department of Health, put forward the clearest explication of the Minister's thinking on nursing policy when he addressed a meeting of the Irish Nurses' Organisation in October 1949. Dr Deeny outlined the reasons for the introduction of the legislation put forward by Dr Browne. The Nurses Bill was introduced on the basis of 'many and weighty' factors, including factors of national concern and factors relating to the nursing profession and the training of nurses.[18] Dr Deeny pointed to the disparity between the nation's needs for a nursing service and the absence of the State's prerogative in the recruitment and training of nurses:

> For various reasons it has become an established fact that this country maintains training schools for the nursing profession – that nurses are trained, but that the training of nurses could not be said to be properly related to national needs. Nurses are trained here but once they are trained they may vanish from the country to the four ends of the earth. Neither the General Nursing Council nor anyone else has power or authority to train a nurse or group of nurses for any special work or post. For instance … if Dr Browne decides that he will open a new Orthopaedic Hospital, say in two years, he cannot go to the Central Nursing Council (*sic*) and say to them that he wants a nursing staff trained for such a hospital. If he did, the General Nursing Council would have no powers to assist him.[19]

The lack of a national perspective in the recruitment and training of nurses was at variance with the Government's plans for developing a comprehensive national health service. This state of affairs could not be permitted to continue, given that there was 'a national need to relate the training of nurses to the needs of this country's hospitals and public health services'.

The new regulatory authority proposed in the Nurses Bill would be known as An Bord Altranais (the Nursing Board); it would have responsibility for the training of nurses and midwives and it would also have the bigger picture of the nation's needs in mind. The new authority could also arrange research into the work of nurses, in order to examine and, if appropriate, apply new understandings concerning the efficiency of nurses' work. The existing training schools would continue to play a role in the training of nurses and it was not the intention of the Minister to 'interfere with their internal arrangements'. A training school with a good record in providing well-trained nurses could expect help and assistance rather than interference from the new Nursing Board.

It was also anticipated that the new Nursing Board would play a more active role in developing and delivering training programmes for nurses and midwives, and would be in a position to initiate and be responsible for special training courses for 'district health work', or for higher posts, including teachers of nursing. Given the advances in nursing, including increased clinical specialization, nursing needed to 'be revitalised by a unifying process' and the constitution of a new regulatory authority would achieve this. In view of the need to give greater prominence to the public health aspects of nursing, Dr Deeny called for more instruction in subjects such as hygiene, sociology, preventive medicine, psychology, and educational methods. The curriculum should also afford nurses the opportunity to study a 'hobby subject', such as English, music, painting or dressmaking. The Nurses Bill would permit a new and more flexible approach to the training of nurses and it would permit nursing to play 'even a greater part in the life of the Nation'.

While the Irish Nurses' Organisation had reservations concerning the establishment of separate disciplinary procedures for nurses and midwives and reservations concerning the capacity of the proposed legislation to safeguard the title 'Registered Nurse', it welcomed the Nurses Bill.[20] Senator Bigger, the former Chairman of the General Nursing Council, also welcomed the bill, but he too had reservations.[21] He considered the powers that the bill conferred on the Minister for Health to be too great and he expressed concern that the new Nursing Board could establish its own training school, a prospect that he considered to be undesirable. The correct function of the new Board, he argued, was to arrange the curriculum and examinations and deal with registration and the question of discipline. Despite the reservations, the Nurses Bill was not contentious in the party political sense and its passage through the Dáil and Senate was relatively quick.[22]

The Nursing Board and regulation of training

The Nurses Act 1950 dissolved the General Nursing Council for Ireland and the Central Midwives Board and it established the Nursing Board. In establishing a single regulatory authority for nursing and midwifery, the Act effectively sub-sumed the title 'midwife' under the title 'nurse'.[23] The new authority was constituted with a membership of twenty-three, to include ten registered nurses elected by nurses from the principal branches of nursing and midwifery, and thir-teen ministerial appointees, including six medical persons, one educator, two representatives from local government, and two registered nurses. The Board's term of office was five years, and it was empowered to elect a President, to appoint officers and servants, to establish committees, and to draw up rules.

The General Nursing Council for Ireland was formally dissolved on 21 February 1951 and the new Nursing Board was formally constituted at its first meeting on 7 June 1951.[24] Opening the first meeting of the Board, An Taoiseach (Prime Minister) John A. Costello paid tribute to the work of the outgoing regula-tory bodies and he welcomed the members of the new Nursing Board, expressing confidence that the Board 'would carry out its functions with zeal and effi-ciency'.[25] The new Board elected Dr Patrick MacCarville, the outgoing Chairman of the General Nursing Council, as its first President. At the Board's first meeting, Dr MacCarville set out the Board's policy. He declared that if it was the intention of the Nurses Act to revolutionize nursing in Ireland, then he was not in favour of that, and he cautioned that the changes intended by the Act should be made in a conservative way. The functions of the Nurses Act were to provide improvements in nurse training and to provide the public health nurses that were needed for the health services. While the training of nurses 'wanted improvements', Dr MacCarville believed that 'Irish trained nurses were the best in the world, and the excellent training they received … was [due to] the contri-bution of the Irish doctor, the Irish tutor and the Irish matron'.[26]

The Nursing Board appointed Mr James Keogh as Chief Executive Officer in 1952, and in 1955 it appointed Roseanne Cunningham, a former nurse tutor at St Vincent's Hospital and the Children's Hospital Temple Street, as Education Officer.[27] It established committees, including the Finance Committee, the Midwives Committee, the Rules Committee and a Committee on Outdoor Nursing Services. The Rules Committee prepared draft Nurses Rules, which the Board approved and published in 1953. *The Nurses Rules 1953* set out the role and functions of the Board in relation to the Register of Nurses, the approval of train-ing hospitals and institutions, the duration of training, and the conduct of examinations.[28]

Under the *Nurses Rules*, hospitals or institutions seeking approval as training institutions were required to submit an application for approval, along with 'a full description of its training material, [and] the amount of training experience each nurse is assured'. Institutions were also required to give evidence 'of educational facilities and of the existence of systematic arrangements whereby the attendance of each training nurse at a series of lectures on the prescribed subjects is assured.' The standard of nursing care in an applying institution could be taken as evi-dence in the approval process and each institution was required to make available student living accommodation 'of a satisfactory standard'. The Board could inspect an institution in advance of giving approval and from time to time.

The *Nurses Rules* also set down the normal periods of training, stipulating three years as the period for all registration programmes, except Midwives and Infectious Diseases Nurses, the periods for which were set at two years. Provision was also made for shortened periods of training to permit registered nurses to undertake a further period of training, normally of two years' duration, to gain entry to a second division of the Register.[29] The Infectious Diseases Nurses Division and the Sanatorium Nurses Division later became redundant, owing to the decline in tuberculosis and other infectious diseases, and two new divisions, the Mental Handicap and Public Health Nurses divisions, were later added. While the *Nurses Rules* did not set down minimum educational requirements for entry to nursing, the matron of each hospital was required to interview the candidate and advise the Board as to his/her suitability.

In 1955, the Board issued *Regulations and Guides* as to the minimum conditions that should exist before a hospital or institution could receive approval as a training institution.[30] The *Regulations and Guides* established minimum standards relating to clinical and teaching facilities and personnel, student accommodation and student welfare. A hospital seeking approval as a general training hospital should have a minimum of one hundred beds, with a wide range of clinical departments, including medicine, surgery, out-patient or casualty department, an operating theatre, X-ray and physiotherapy departments, and have consultants and adequate numbers of resident medical staff. Minimum teaching facilities should include a properly equipped lecture room to seat the entire body of students, a study room, a practice room, a diet kitchen and a library with up-to-date textbooks and nursing periodicals. The provision of a 'simple laboratory' and a sister tutor's office was recommended. Personnel should be available to participate in the instruction of students, including a medical practitioner with a diploma in public health, a professor or lecturer in surgery, a dietician, an almoner, a pharmacist and a minister of religion. Nursing personnel should include a matron, a sister tutor and 'adequate numbers' of staff nurses and ward sisters. The *Regulations and Guides* prescribed minimum nurse–patient ratios of one staff nurse to fifteen patients and one student nurse to five patients, while the teacher–student ratio should be one sister tutor to forty students. Institutions seeking approval should provide a separate bedroom for each student and adequate recreation facilities. Students should also be given a medical examination, including a chest X-ray and a Mantoux test, and have immunization against diphtheria and regular chest X-rays during training.

Compliance with the *Regulations and Guides* would ensure that the nurse in training received broad and varied clinical experiences, reflecting the range of clinical cases and clinical activities occurring in a modern hospital. The requirements pertaining to nurses' living and health arrangements maintained the student nurse in the custodianship of the hospital and reflected her continued material importance.

Instruction and the role of the nurse

The Nursing Board's *Syllabus of Courses of Instruction* set out the theoretical and clinical instruction required for the first, second and third years of general training.[31] The syllabus for the first year prescribed lectures in elementary anatomy and physiology, first aid, hygiene, invalid cookery, and theory and practice of nursing. Instruction should also include history of nursing, ethics of nursing, hospital etiquette, hospital economy, domestic ward management, and the observation and care of the sick. The syllabus for the second and third years prescribed lectures in bacteriology, dietetics, materia medica, medicine, surgery, gynaecology, eye and ear, and theory and practice of nursing. It was recommended that the lectures in hygiene and bacteriology should be taken early in the course and that 'particular attention should be paid to those matters which are of every-day practical use to the Nurse while tending the sick'. Emphasis was placed on the relative importance of practical competence in learning the theory and practice of nursing:

> It is more important that the Nurse should be able to recognize those symptoms and signs which indicate the onset of trouble than that they should be conversant with the pathology of the disease … In the description of the various diseases particular attention should be paid to matters which will assist the Nurse in the observation of symptoms, and in the care of the patient.[32]

The syllabus also prescribed the methods and organization of instruction. Teaching methods should include lectures, discussions, experiments, demonstrations, tutorials, the use of audio-visual aids, and visits to places of interest, and reference was made to:

> (a) the importance of giving the student an understanding of the principles rather than unnecessary depth in subject matter; (b) allowing adequate time for study; (c) the value of the study day or half study day during the early part of her training; (d) the advantage of using, in the second and third years, the partial block system.[33]

While clinical instruction was not prescribed in the precise way that theoretical instruction was, the syllabus implied the sort of duties that the nurse in training was expected to perform.[34] In the first year, the duties of the student nurse included domestic ward management, general care of the patient, the recording of physical signs, the administration of medicines, and the application of dressings. During the second and third years, the student nurse provided nursing care to persons with a range of medical and surgical conditions, and her duties included observing and recording signs and symptoms, administering medicines, managing symptoms, and caring for persons undergoing surgical operations. The syllabus implied that the student would develop a range of generic and specific nursing skills in a variety of clinical departments and that these skills would be transferred across the care of many and varied clinical cases.

The syllabus did not reflect the sort of nursing role envisaged by the Minister for Health when he introduced the Nurses Bill in 1949; while Dr Browne believed that nurses' training should equip them to work in the 'preventive side of public health', the syllabus implied that they would continue to work in the setting of the hospital ward.[35] The original and primary intention of the Nurses Act was to procure the rational recruitment and training of nurses in order to meet the projected needs of an expanding public health service during the 1950s and beyond. In 1949, the total number of nurses enrolled on the General Nursing Council's Register was 6,736, of which more than two-thirds (4,536) were general nurses.[36] A decade later, the number of general nurses had risen to 8,525, an effective doubling of the number.[37] However, the Register of Nurses did not yet contain a division for public health nurses.

In 1959, thirty approved hospitals were providing general nurse training in Ireland.[38] In 1960, the Nursing Board established the Diploma for Nurse Tutors in association with University College Dublin, thereby introducing formal training for teachers of nursing. During the mid-1970s, the Board approved a new combined four-year general and sick children's nurse training programme at a number of Dublin hospitals, and it also approved a combined four-year general and psychiatric nurse training programme.[39] While nurses and midwives were strongly represented on the Board, the Minister for Health had the authority to directly appoint the Board's President.[40] In all but the final year of its first thirty years, a medical practitioner held the post of President of the Board. In 1979, Charles Haughey, the then Minister for Health, appointed Joan Barlow as the first nurse President of the Board.

Conditions of employment

After 1950, the *Nurses Rules* 1953, the *Syllabus of Courses of Instruction*, and the *Regulations and Guides* determined much of what the student nurse experienced in her training. However, as obtaining in the period before 1950, the student nurse's curricular experiences were determined by her role as a hospital worker and by her conditions of employment. During the Senate debate on the Nurses Bill of 1949, a number of Senators raised concerns regarding nurses' conditions of employment. Nurses' remuneration, their enduring difficulties in procuring a pension scheme, and the poor quality of nurses' accommodation were highlighted, and nurses' conditions of employment, including accommodation and recreational facilities, were cited as a reason for the difficulties in recruiting and retaining nurses.[41]

A subsidiary aim of the Nurses Bill was the improvement in nurses' living arrangements, and some improvements were effected when the Minister for Health Dr Ryan opened new nurses' homes at St Michael's Hospital in 1951, and at the Meath and the Incorporated Orthopaedic hospitals in 1952.[42] Dr Ryan's successor T. F. O'Higgins performed the same task at the Mater Misericordiae Hospital in 1954, opening a facility containing 231 separate bedrooms for nurses and sisters.[43]

The construction of a large stock of nurses' accommodation in the period meant that the nurses' home remained as an enduring feature of the training experience under the new Nursing Board. Hospitals continued to maintain a custodial function in relation to student nurses; the Minister for Health Dr Browne acknowledged this in 1950, remarking that 'these girls are young girls, and the officers in these institutions act in *loco parentis*'.[44] However, Dr Browne expressed concern at the regime of tight control operating in nurses' homes and he called on hospitals to adopt 'a more liberal attitude in the matter of recreation, discipline and the comings and goings generally of nurses'.

While the training period was nominally of three years' duration, many hospitals operated an arrangement by which the student was obligated to give a fourth year of 'experience' in the service of her training hospital. While she received her registration status after three years, she continued to receive the salary of a third-year student nurse and was not granted her hospital badge or hospital diploma until she completed the fourth year.[45] This 'staying on' period was presented to the student as recompense to her hospital for the training that she received.[46] The Minister for Health Donogh O'Malley disapproved of the arrangement, and in 1966 he called on hospitals to abandon the practice.[47] While some voluntary hospitals argued that the additional year was necessary in view of the considerable educational needs of the student, the 'staying on' period was afterwards abandoned.[48]

Instruction and pedagogy

In 1960, the Nursing Board introduced the requirement that a preliminary training school was an essential condition for approval as a training hospital. While many institutions were operating a preliminary training school at the time, the requirement ensured that all students received a protected period of theoretical instruction before they entered the hospital wards. The period of instruction ranged from eight to twelve weeks.[49] The preliminary training school did not merely function to prepare the student for her first clinical placement and her first State examinations, but it also introduced her to the organization's culture and to her place in the organizational structure. At St Vincent's Hospital in the late 1950s, the preliminary training school introduced the student to the hospital way of life:

> Here she is gently and gradually initiated into the pattern of her new life … and is equipped to adapt herself to this new [ward] environment with greater ease to herself, and less risk to her patients … She starts on the course specified for Anatomy and Physiology … She is taken to see an operation in progress. This is one of the highlights of her stay in the preliminary training school, an opportunity which she might not expect for one or two years in the ordinary course of training. She is initiated gently into the discipline required for nurses, and happily is shown first the necessity for discipline.[50]

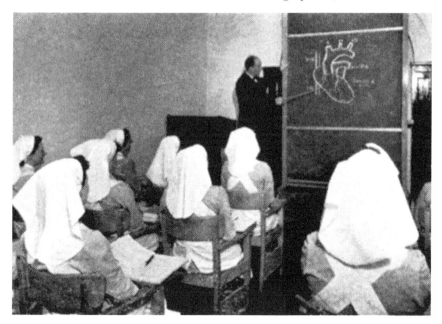

Figure 7.1 In block, St Vincent's Hospital, Dublin, 1957. Courtesy of St Vincent's University Hospital, Dublin

In its operation, the preliminary training school had implied functions related to the professional socialization of the nurse, and research conducted by Simpson in the 1960s pointed to its function of inculcating professional values:

> [In the preliminary training school] student nurses are required to wear uniform, to be punctual for lectures, to hand in lecture notes for inspection, to refer to one another as 'nurse' and to comply with regulations about personal belongings, behaviour and use of school premises. It is expected that this externally imposed discipline will carry over onto the ward.[51]

The training hospital was a micro community, comprising individuals and groups, and each individual occupied a particular place in the hospital hierarchy. While in the preliminary training school, the 'PTS' student occupied the lowest position in this hierarchy; because hospital domestics were often highly valued members of the staff, they could enjoy a high degree of power on the ward and the PTS had to know her place in this arrangement.[52] The 'graduation' from PTS to second-year student was an important milestone in the life of the student nurse; at the Adelaide Hospital, this graduation was symbolized by changing from PTS caps 'to the glamorous ones with five pleats'.[53]

In response to a recommendation of the Nursing Board and the Minister for Health Donogh O'Malley in 1966, most training hospitals introduced the 'block' system.[54] Like the preliminary training school, the system provided uninterrupted periods of lectures and replaced the ad hoc arrangements whereby students

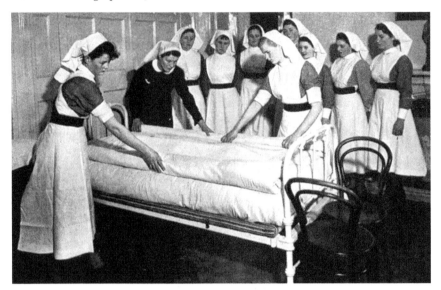

Figure 7.2 In the practical room, St Vincent's Hospital, Dublin, 1957. Courtesy of St
Vincent's University Hospital, Dublin

attended lectures in their off-duty periods. The Nursing Board recommended a
total of eighteen to twenty-two weeks of block instruction over the three years, to
include eight to ten weeks in the first year, and two periods of five to six weeks, in
each of the second and third years. Mr O'Malley viewed the block system as
desirable, since it made it easier for the student to 'assimilate the instruction she is
receiving and at the same time avoid the disruption of nursing services which
arises when a student has to switch back and forth between ward duties and lectures'.[55] The system provided a programme of structured teaching and planned
assessments and permitted the recruitment of students on a twice-yearly basis.[56]
Students welcomed the block system, since it gave them temporary relief from
their commitments to ward work and it ended the requirement to attend lectures
during their off-duty time.[57] Reflecting the position of the student nurse as a hospital worker, the block system was generally planned according to the particular
needs of each individual hospital.

While the majority of training schools were operating the block system by
1970, some matrons were finding it impossible to operate a full or even a partial
block system because of staff shortages, and a small number of Dublin hospitals
continued to operate a system of morning and evening lectures.[58] In addition,
some student nurses were required to work on the wards while examinations were
in session and were permitted to be absent from duty only when they were sched-
uled to sit for their examinations. As late as 1972, a number of hospitals were
failing to operate the requisite preliminary training period and some did not pay
student nurses during the preliminary training period.[59]

Aside from the variance in the ways that instruction was organized, there was
also considerable variance among the hospitals in the proportion of time that they

each allotted to individual subjects.[60] Some nursing schools were providing instruction well in excess of the Nursing Board's prescribed minimum periods while others were failing to meet the minimum requirements, and some schools were failing to provide prescribed instruction in the biological sciences, the social sciences, and 'social aspects of nursing'.[61] Many schools also lacked resources for teaching, including adequate library resources. In a more general sense, the curriculum was considered to be deficient in a number of key areas, and in the early 1960s, a World Health Organization (WHO) Expert Committee on Nursing called for teaching in 'prevention and social, as well as curative nursing content'.[62] In 1962, through its President Miss F. O'Sullivan, the Public Health Nurses Section of the Irish Nurses' Organisation questioned the extent to which the basic nursing curriculum in Ireland paid adequate attention to 'social, physical and environmental indices of health'.[63] Concern was also expressed that there was no provision for obstetrical experience in the general nursing curriculum, 'a marked deficiency' that prevented many registered nurses from taking up positions abroad.[64]

While there was variance in the amount of time given to individual subjects across institutions, by the 1970s new subjects were appearing. These included social medicine, community health, care of the terminal patient, geriatrics, psychiatry, and physics and chemistry.[65] Curriculum innovation tended to occur organically, whereby new subjects and new pedagogical methods were introduced in individual schools by individual nurse tutors.[66] There was greater use of 'modern teaching methods', such as the group discussion, a method that one sister tutor recommended, since it trained the young student 'to think, to learn to express herself, to have the courage to put forward her own views, and above all to accept criticism'.[67] While the benefits of 'modern teaching methods' were recognized, extolling their use might have been more rhetoric than any real commitment to them. Evidence from Hanrahan's survey conducted among student nurses in the Dublin hospitals in the late 1960s hinted that the pedagogical reality of the classroom was one in which group discussions were rarely used, lectures were often presented as 'crash courses', and little time was provided for private study.[68] Student nurses were dissatisfied that lecturers were not good at lecturing and that procedures taught in classrooms could not be applied to the ward situation.

The assessment of learning was conducted primarily through written and oral examinations. Oral and 'practical' examinations were conducted by medical and surgical consultants and by hospital matrons. As a component of the Final Examination set by the Nursing Board, the oral examination complemented the written part and it functioned to assess the student in her knowledge of medicine, surgery, pharmacology, pathology and nursing. The oral examinations assumed enormous importance for student nurses and many dreaded the ordeal.[69]

On the wards

Aside from the instruction received in the preliminary training school and in block, learning on the wards was the other major part of the student nurse's

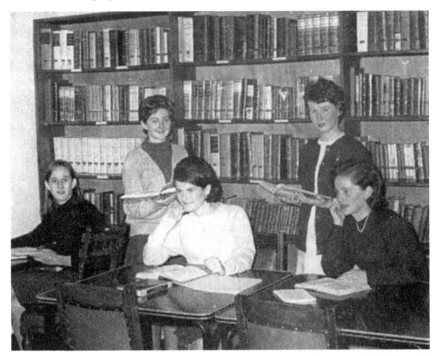

Figure 7.3 In the library, St Vincent's Hospital, Dublin, 1964. Courtesy of St Vincent's University Hospital, Dublin

curricular experience. Learning on the wards meant working on the wards, and the student nurse could expect to work up to ninety-six hours a fortnight.[70] Many hospitals operated a 'split' duty system, which effectively required the student to work two duty-shifts in a single day.

Writing about the system of apprenticeship nurse training in British hospitals during the 1960s, Bradshaw remarked:

> A hundred years after nurse training began at the Nightingale School, there is every indication that Nightingale's principles still dominated British nursing. The ward sister still controlled the ward in which the student nurse learned … Specified nursing work included giving bowls and mouthwashes, attention to pressure areas, feeding seriously ill patients, charting fluids, recording observations, and performing nursing treatments. Each task had a prescribed time, which included a time for ward prayers.[71]

Based on the planning and completion of routine tasks, this system of work characterized the way that hospital wards functioned. Tasks and procedures tended to become ends in themselves and the student nurse was a key participant in the everyday routine of this task-oriented work. The British nurse's counterpart in the Irish hospital ward underwent a similar experience that included the routines of 'damp dusting and bed pan rounds'.[72]

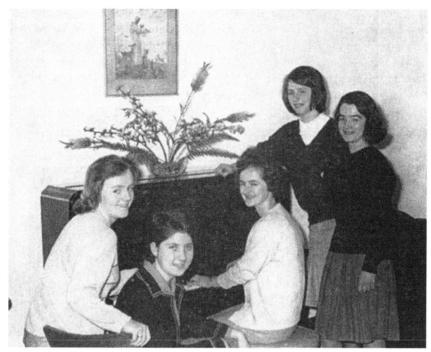

Figure 7.4 In the nurses' home, St Vincents' Hospital, Dublin, 1964. Courtesy of St Vincent's University Hospital, Dublin

The experience of learning on the wards included the first day on the wards, an event of great significance in the life of the student nurse. Although frightening, in retrospect, the experience tended to be remembered with fondness.[73] Despite her lack of experience, the student nurse was given much responsibility for the care of patients; while on night duty, it was not unusual for a student nurse to take charge of a ward and to carry out duties for which she was not adequately trained.[74] However, a great part of her duties were related to hospital household work, and one nurse who trained at the Adelaide Hospital during the 1960s remarked with irony on the contrast between the ideal and the reality of nurse training:

> have you never realized how privileged we who trained in the old days actually were, from the first day that we were handed our wooden boxes and sent to clean the bathrooms. A symbol of disillusionment those boxes, nothing like them to wipe the virtuous smile off the face of an innocent eighteen year old. Never again would we have highfalutin' ideas about vocations, or even the alleviation of suffering, we just took out the Ajax and got on with it.[75]

Learning on the wards meant learning on the job and planned clinical teaching was a limited activity, owing partly to the insufficient supply of clinical teachers to meet the demands of student training.[76] Moreover, most of the training hospitals had fewer than 250 beds, thereby limiting the range of experiences available to the student.[77] Nevertheless, each student was required to complete a list of 'practical nursing procedures and other duties appropriate to the care of the patient' before being permitted to enter for the State examinations.[78] On completion of each ward placement, the student's progress was checked against the list of procedures in her procedure book and a report of her progress was submitted to the matron.[79] Introduced in the 1950s by the Nursing Board as a means of ascertaining if a student had attained proficiency, the procedure book contained a record of instruction given in such areas as 'administration of medicines' and 'ward dressings'.

The student nurse's experiences of learning on the wards were moderated by the perceived and actual tension between her role as a learner and a worker, and this tension could be part of her curricular experience.[80] Despite the prevailing threat to learning, student nurses valued ward learning over classroom learning and held the role of worker as pre-eminent over that of student.[81]

Living in and 'the set'

An abiding feature of the training experience was the proliferation of rules that governed the student nurse's life and work, and nowhere were these rules more prevalent than in relation to living in the nurses' home. The majority of student nurses resided in the nurses' home during their training, and they worked and recreated together for the most part. Life in the nurses' home at the Mater Misericordiae Hospital was described in 1961:

> The College [of Nursing] offers the most modern and up to date residence for student nurses and every amenity for pleasant living … [and] life in the College is very pleasant for students. There is of course the discipline which is essential for any student if she is to benefit from her studies. Otherwise there is … a true spirit of friendliness and good fellowship.[82]

This description of an idyll of 'pleasant living' also contains reference to two of the enduring features of life in the nurses' home, namely the regime of discipline and the companionship that existed amongst the students. In the 1960s, discipline was still viewed as a necessary part of the training of the nurse:

> A student nurse's life is essentially one of discipline, a never ending series of acts of self-renunciation … she is in need of much direction and guidance if she is to breach successfully the gap from immaturity to the acceptance of serious responsibility for the welfare of the sick … [Discipline] is absolutely necessary for the student nurse if she is to make a success of her profession.[83]

Most young women had entered nursing from a secondary school system that encouraged conformity to rules, and nurse training represented a continuation of this type of system.[84] Strict rules governed the wearing of the nurse's uniform; the daily uniform inspection by the matron or the sister tutor was a ritual in many hospitals. Students' comings and goings were monitored and controlled and recreation was frequently organized on a group basis, usually under the auspices of the hospital social club. Students participated in a variety of group activities, such as carol singing at Christmas, nurses' dances, swimming and other social outings. Hospitals provided recreational facilities, including tennis, table tennis, television and radio, and a record player.

The student nurse's experience on first entering the nurses' home was a portent of future experiences. For one student nurse who commenced her training at St Vincent's Hospital in 1956, her first impressions of the nurses' home was of a building with 'a lovely old world atmosphere', while her counterpart who commenced training at the Mater Misericordiae Hospital in the early 1960s experienced 'the most modern and up to date [nurses'] residence'.[85] While the nurses' home could be opulent, it could also be austere. One nurse who trained at the Adelaide Hospital in the 1950s recalls the 'cultural shock' of moving into 'a large unheated building, bare of furnishing apart from the half curtains on the windows'.[86] In the nurses' home, she was required to check in at 9.15 pm and was granted a late pass until midnight once a month. With such restrictions, student nurses frequently flouted the rules and took risks by 'escaping' at night; in making good their escape, student nurses at the Adelaide Hospital made use of the fire escape or the laundry basket.[87] This flouting of the rules was a part of what it meant to be a student nurse, and in her research into student life in 1968, Simpson wrote:

> groups of eighteen year old student nurses isolated in the preliminary training school take a delight in contravening minor restrictions. If the front door is locked at night, then it is fun to climb in through the window after hours. If silence is imposed in private study periods, then it is fun to talk.[88]

Hospitals discouraged student nurses from living out and required them to reside in the nurses' home during the first and second years of training. While the nurses' home provided secure and inexpensive accommodation and the companionship of fellow students, it did not satisfy the desire on the part of many students for a social life away from 'the hospital atmosphere'.[89]

In 1966, having considered the restrictions placed on the student nurse, the Minister for Health Donogh O'Malley prepared a series of recommendations on the training conditions of student nurses. The Minister called on all institutions involved in nurse training to allow 'the maximum freedom consistent, of course, with their ages, [and] the expressed wishes of their parents'.[90] He called on institutions to realistically examine the hours at which student nurses were required to return to the nurses' home 'in the light of the prevailing standards for girls' corresponding age and status'. Despite the Minister's wishes, the restrictive custodial regime, including the requirement to 'check-in', persisted in many general training schools in the 1970s and, in some instances, into the 1980s.

While the student nurse was a member of the hospital community, with its own values, traditions and culture, she was also a member of the general body of student nurses, and within that body, she belonged to her 'set'. The set was the student's training group and, along with giving each student her identity within the organization, membership of her set conferred certain benefits, including companionship during training and lifelong friendships:

> [At the Adelaide Hospital] twenty of us had started our training together in August 1971. There were to be many more funny, difficult and sad times during our years in the Adelaide, but all these shared experiences, the excellent teaching we received and our everyday work together, established a strong team spirit, and made for many lifelong friendships.[91]

The set had important social and symbolic functions and it also had the features and functions of a sub-culture. Students of the same set tended to recreate together and, as a locus of companionship, the set established group identity for its members and reinforced group solidarity.[92] From a review of studies undertaken into nurse training in Britain in the 1960s, Simpson provided a description of the set, its functions and its dysfunctions:

> Students start hospital life as a group or set and build up strong relationships based on the 'set'. The hierarchical nature of the hospital social structure reinforces their interdependence of members of the set and so does the constant change of ward, which, whilst necessary as a training experience, prevents team consciousness developing in the work situation. Students then are much dependent on other members of their set for companionship and for support when difficulties arise. This can make for loneliness when the set are split up between different hospitals and even as a result of the different off duty times which inevitably fall to the various members of the set.[93]

The set also delineated status positions within the student body and, as MacGuire noted, 'the hierarchy of the sets within the grade of student nurse in a hospital, constitutes the sum total of the various status positions which are available'.[94] In this way, the set not only denoted the individual student's status vis-à-vis other students, but it placed limits on her mobility within the hierarchy:

> the principle on which the sets are stratified is occupational skill … Mobility in the system is based on the principle of 'social age' – that is the length of time the individual student nurse has been associated with the hospital. Mobility is group not individual based. Seniority is reckoned not in years, but in intervals between intakes, no allowance is made for chronological age, maturity, experience or response to training.[95]

While student nurses in Ireland were beginning to form student associations and had begun to establish affiliations with the newly formed Student Nurses Section of the Irish Nurses' Organisation, the set persisted with its symbolic role in establishing status positions and its practical role in procuring companionship.

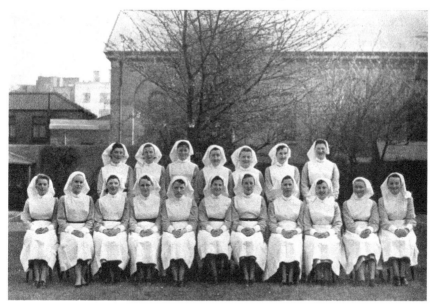

Figure 7.5 The set, third-year student nurses, St. Vincent's Hospital, Dublin, 1957.
Courtesy of St Vincent's University Hospital, Dublin

Recruitment

In Ireland during the 1950s and 1960s, emigration was a constant and nursing was not immune to this social phenomenon. Throughout this period, many nurses left Ireland on completion of their training because of the lack of opportunities for employment at home, the lure of wider experience and career opportunities abroad, and the call to do missionary work.[96] Many nurses emigrated to England where they could find better conditions of employment. While retention of staff was a problem for many hospitals, the large voluntary hospitals in Dublin and in the other major cities had little difficulty recruiting student nurses. Nursing remained an attractive career choice for young middle-class women, and many hospitals had waiting lists for a place in training.[97] Nursing provided salaried employment and a professional training at a time when the Irish economy was relatively small, when few parents could afford a university education for their children, and when there were limited alternative career opportunities for young women.[98]

By the late 1960s, the profile of the women recruited to nursing in the Dublin hospitals indicated that the majority were drawn from rural areas, this trend being consistent with the wider phenomenon of rural-urban migration then prevalent in Ireland.[99] The majority of recruits were school leavers who had attended Catholic-administered secondary schools and had attained Leaving Certificate honours or pass standard. Relative to other countries, recruits to nursing in Ireland had a high standard of secondary education; the fact that the majority had attained the Leaving Certificate standard of education suggests that nursing was not the only career choice open to them. For many recruits, nursing was their

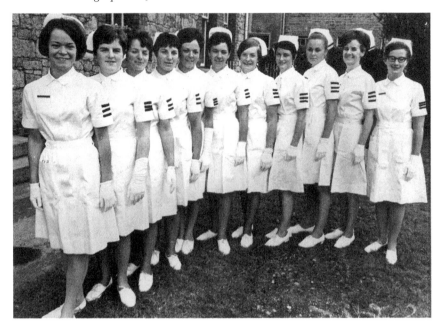

Figure 7.6 First set, School of Nursing, St James's Hospital, Dublin, *c.*1968. Courtesy of St
     James's Hospital, Dublin

first and only career choice and most made multiple applications to hospitals in an
effort to secure a place in nurse training. While parents of the recruits to nursing
approved of their daughters' career choice, their teachers were less inclined to
encourage them to pursue nursing as a career.[100]

In the 1970s, recruitment patterns continued to reflect the popularity of nursing as a career for young educated women of school-leaving age. Despite the low
salaries and the limited promotional opportunities, recruitment remained high
and wastage was relatively low.[101] For example, in 1975, the Royal City of Dublin
Hospital received 2,500 applications for the thirty training places available.[102]
While the Nursing Board did not specify it as the minimum educational requirement for entry to nurse training, the Leaving Certificate had effectively become
the minimum entry requirement by the early 1970s and many hospitals were giving preference to students who presented with mathematics and one or more of
the basic sciences.[103] Recruitment from the male population was low; most of the
males entering general nurse training were nurses on the Psychiatric and Mental
Handicap divisions of the Register seeking preparation for the General division,
and it was only in the late 1970s that men were increasingly admitted directly to
general nurse training.[104]

Commentary on the system of training

The better qualities of the training system in Ireland were considered to be a
function of the good personal qualities that were developed in the Irish nurse,

who was regarded as 'a concerned, competent and skilful practitioner who gives excellent nursing care'.[105] In addition, students tended to develop strong bonds with their training hospital, and many reciprocated for the professional training that they received by taking up positions as staff nurses and by maintaining a strong sense of loyalty to the hospital.[106]

Despite these admirable features, international thinking on the training of nurses held that it should be conducted as an enterprise separate from nursing service. In 1955, a WHO study group called for full student status for the student nurse and a broad-based curriculum that prepared the nurse for her responsibilities not only towards the ill person but also towards the healthy.[107] Later, in 1973, a WHO representative expressed concern that the training of nurses had 'little relevance to present or future professional requirements' and remarked:

> the dependence of hospitals on student nurses to provide 60–80% of the nursing services shows how illusory the educational experience is since under these circumstances learning becomes centred on the technical and routine aspects of care.[108]

International commentators also questioned the extent to which hospital schools of nursing could ever function as educational institutions. At the Congress of the International Council of Nurses in 1968, one commentator observed that the hospital school of nursing was an anachronism, since the aims of education could not be met where the student's time was controlled by the service needs of the hospital.[109]

In Ireland, too, there were concerns about the quality of nurse training. It was contended that student nurses merely repeated nursing routines, that learning was not incrementally planned, and that students could be given duties beyond their capability.[110] There were also calls for the elimination of the 'rigid discipline and regimentation' in nurse training and their replacement with a 'human approach' and with new pedagogical strategies.[111] In her analysis of the system of apprenticeship nurse training in Ireland, which she undertook in the early 1960s, Pauline Scanlan concluded that the most fundamental criticism of basic nurse training in Ireland was that there was 'not one programme conducted under an educational authority'.[112] Scanlan highlighted the fact that recruits to nursing were being admitted for training on eleven out of the twelve months of the year. This practice ran counter to the State's policy of a more rational approach to the recruitment and training of nurses; individual institutions were recruiting solely with reference to their own local service needs.

Despite these concerns, it was recognized that few Irish hospitals could operate without the services provided by the labour of student nurses.[113] The Nursing Board recognized the limits of its statutory powers in respect of the nursing service in each training hospital, conceding that the selection of students was the responsibility of each hospital and acknowledging the great impact that any new training arrangements would have on the training hospitals.[114]

Conclusions

The Nurses Act of 1950 was introduced on the premise that nurses and midwives would be recruited rationally and trained adequately to play their part in developing and delivering the health services that were projected to expand. Despite initiatives to develop community health services, the independent voluntary hospital continued to be the locus for the delivery of a large part of the health services to the population. With an increasing array of specialist technical medical services, the hospital had further consolidated its position as the dominant model of publicly funded health care. Within the hospital, the nurse in training continued to play a key role in providing the services, and the Nursing Board's *Syllabus of Courses of Instruction* seemed to confirm the pre-eminence of the nurse's role as a hospital nurse.

Throughout its first thirty years, the Nursing Board fulfilled its statutory mandate to regulate nursing and midwifery. By the mid-1970s, approximately 1000 nurses were registered annually and the Nursing Board enabled improvements and updating of training programmes.[115] The Board was responsive to developments in nursing and healthcare, revising the syllabus from time to time, facilitating the widening of clinical learning experiences, and facilitating some curriculum innovation.[116] Overall, however, the first thirty years of the Board's tenure were characterized by relative stability in nursing and in the nursing curriculum.

Although derived from the statutory provisions set out in the *Syllabus of Courses of Instruction* and the *Regulations and Guides*, the student nurse's curricular experiences were mediated by local interpretations of these provisions, by pragmatic imperatives related to the student's position as a hospital employee, and by the organizational structure and milieu of her training hospital. Writing on the training of nurses in 1957, Sister Francis Rose, a tutor sister at St Vincent's Hospital, observed:

> the curriculum in a school of nursing is planned so that each student develops her own individuality, whilst at the same time certain characteristics must be deepened and others subdued.[117]

Pedagogical relationships and the entire range of curricular experiences appear to have been predicated upon this general premise. Characteristics were either deepened or subdued in and through the range of experiences presented to the student in the preliminary training school, in block, on the wards, and in the nurses' home.

Throughout the decades 1950 to 1980, nurses lobbied for improved conditions of employment, and in the 1970s they achieved some success when they procured a substantial increase in salary. The state of the national economy was a significant factor in determining nurses' conditions of employment and it was the most significant factor in ensuring that the student nurse would remain as a hospital employee. Despite international calls for the separation of nurse training from nursing service, the student nurse remained an essential resource in the delivery of the hospital-based health services.

8 From the hospital to the academy, 1980–1994

The 1980s was a decade of transition for nurse training in Ireland. At the start of the decade, the system of hospital apprenticeship training was secure as an integral part of hospital nursing, and the student nurse remained as an essential resource in the delivery of the hospital-based health services. By the decade's end, the system was much less secure and its future sustainability was being undermined by professional and educational imperatives and by new economic realities.

Nursing policy in the 1980s

In the 1980s, Irish Government health policy was articulated in the consultative document *Health – the Wider Dimensions*.[1] Published in 1986, the document endorsed the World Health Organization European Region's call for a greater emphasis on preventative approaches in the development of public health services.[2] However, in its proposals concerning the organization of primary healthcare services, the report failed to spell out the role of the nurse and implicitly left medicine in a central role with its cultural values intact and dominant.[3] The policy had little real impact on nursing services or on basic nurse training, and the curriculum continued to emphasize the nurse's role as a hospital nurse. In the period, reduced spending on the health services and long-standing government policy on the re-organization of hospital services in Dublin resulted in a net reduction in the number of hospital beds in the country, but especially in Dublin, where a number of the smaller voluntary hospitals were closed or assimilated into new larger hospitals. Despite this process of rationalization and despite official health policy that called for a re-orientation of the health services towards a health promotion model, the hospital remained dominant in the delivery of public health services, and hospital nursing services continued to be the principal justification for nurse training.

The contribution that nurses were making in the delivery of the health services was widely recognized, but the profession itself was concerned that the nursing role and nursing's future place in the health structures were not clearly defined. The profession was also concerned about staffing structures, communication difficulties between nurses and management, a lack of nursing input into staff planning, deficiencies in the training of nurses, and the impact that anticipated

European Economic Community (EEC) policies would have on nurse training.[4] The Irish Nurses' Organisation, the Irish Matrons' Association and the Nursing Board had each made representations to the Government concerning these matters in the mid 1970s. Following these representations, the then Minister for Health Brendan Corish established a Working Party on General Nursing in 1975. Chaired by Brigid Tierney, a nurse tutor, the Working Party examined the role of nurses in the health service and it considered the education and training requirements for that role. Widely representative of nursing and health service interests, the Working Party presented its Report to the Minister in 1980.

In the most comprehensive examination undertaken of nursing in Ireland to that point, the Working Party presented a total of sixty-six recommendations concerning the role of the nurse, grading structures, recruitment and selection, education and training, and the role of the Nursing Board in the training of nurses. In its report, the Working Party expressed concern about a theory–practice gap in nurse training, which it attributed to the organization of the block system, and it pointed to the lack of standardization in the assessment of learning across training schools. On the basis of these concerns, the Working Party called for the introduction of a modularized system of training, in which theoretical and practical instruction and relevant assessments would be closely related. While the Working Party considered that student nurses could not be totally relieved of their responsibilities in relation to patient care, it argued that the student's commitment to nursing service should not interfere with her educational needs. It also recommended that students be given responsibility for care only in accordance with their level of competence.

The Working Party recommended that a common basic training for all nurses be introduced, consisting of a two-year comprehensive, broad-based programme, followed by one year of intensive training in the student's chosen branch of nursing. Along with proposing a restructuring of the basic training programme, it also proposed an overall reduction in the total number of nurse training schools, and amalgamations of smaller schools. On recruitment and selection, the Working Party called for the establishment of a Central Applications Bureau to operate under the aegis of the Nursing Board, and it recommended that minimum Leaving Certificate entry requirements be established.[5] The Working Party made a number of recommendations concerning the role and functions of the Nursing Board; it called for the introduction of a 'live' register and a register of students, the institution of annual re-registration, and the establishment of a 'fitness to practise' committee. While not ruling out the place of a degree course leading to registration, the Working Party recommended the establishment of a degree course for registered nurses.

Many of the recommendations of the Working Party were contained in the provisions of the Nurses Act of 1985, including recommendations concerning the role of the Nursing Board, the live register, minimum entry requirements, and fitness to practise; the Act effectively established a new Nursing Board, increasing its membership from twenty-three to twenty-nine.[6] The reconstituted Nursing Board was designated as the competent authority to implement any directives on nursing that might emanate from the European Commission and it was also given the responsibility to review and evaluate existing programmes of education and training.[7] In drawing up the Act, the Minister for Health Barry Desmond did not include provision for changes to the structure of nurse training or a reduction in the number of training schools, on the grounds that the Working Party's recommendations in that regard had far-reaching implications that would require further examination.

The European directives

Ireland's membership of the EEC brought considerable prosperity after 1973. With membership, the Irish Government participated in the process of formulating, agreeing and adopting European directives related to economic and social development. While the free movement of labour throughout the member states of the European Community was an important element of the Treaty of Rome, the free movement of professionals required special legislation, in order to assure agreed minimum training standards and permit professionals to practise in any or all of the member states. The development of European directives relating to the mutual recognition of professional qualifications in healthcare became an important expression of the European ideal.[8]

In 1977, a working group of experts from the relevant government departments of the member states submitted new directives on the mutual recognition of nursing qualifications to the European Parliament and these were signed by the Council of Ministers and communicated to the member states on 27 June 1977.[9] Two directives related specifically to 'nurses responsible for general care'. These were Directive 77/452/EEC on the mutual recognition of diplomas or formal qualifications in nursing and Directive 77/453/EEC, which concerned specific requirements for the training programme.[10] On the basis that compliance with European directives should be achieved within two years, the directives became operational in Ireland on 27 June 1979. Responsibility for ensuring compliance was conferred on the Nursing Board.

The European directives afforded Irish nurses enhanced rights in relation to travel and work.[11] In setting down specific requirements for the training programme, including minimum requirements for instruction, Directive 77/453/EEC was of particular importance to the curriculum.[12] The Directive stipulated a three-year course *or* 4,600 hours of theoretical and practical instruction and it stipulated that the theoretical and technical training should be balanced and coordinated with the clinical training.[13] The Annex to the Directive set out a list of subjects to be included in the programme of instruction. Listed under the broad category headings of nursing, basic sciences and social sciences was a range of subjects that included biophysics, biochemistry, sociology, psychology, and social and health legislation. Seven areas of clinical instruction were listed. These were general and specialist medicine, general and specialist surgery, childcare and paediatrics, maternity care, mental health and psychiatry, care of the old and geriatrics, and home nursing.[14]

The training requirements of Directive 77/453/EEC were set out in the Nursing Board's new *Syllabus of Training*.[15] The Nursing Board also issued *Guidelines to the Implementation of the Syllabus of Training*.[16] The Guidelines permitted each training school to plan its own theoretical instruction periods and set down the minimum periods for specialist clinical instruction. Students should receive six weeks of clinical instruction per subject in childcare and paediatrics, mental health and psychiatry, care of the old and geriatrics, accident and emergency/out-patients department, and operating theatre, three weeks in maternity care, and one week in home nursing. The Guidelines also introduced a new assessment structure, comprising the three basic elements of written examinations, oral examinations and clinical assessments. A new method of clinical assessment was introduced, giving individual training hospitals explicit responsibility for assessing students in the development of their clinical skills. The method was based on continuous assessment of a student's clinical learning and incorporated the Proficiency Assessment Form (PAF), which permitted a rating of a student's performance in clinical nursing practice.[17]

With the European directives, schools of nursing began the task of preparing new curricula. Many schools were required either to engage the services of subject specialists in the basic and social sciences or to enter into special arrangements with local technical colleges for the purpose of giving the required instruction. The impact of these new arrangements on hospitals' budgets was negligible when compared with the impact of the new requirements in respect of clinical instruction. While the larger hospitals could provide some specialist clinical instruction, most hospitals were obliged to enter into arrangements with other hospitals for the purpose of providing clinical instruction in paediatrics, psychiatric nursing, geriatric nursing and maternity care. Meeting the requirements of the EEC directives thus presented immediate staffing problems for the training hospitals, since student nurses were unavailable for nursing service for the periods in which they were on 'external' placements.

With the new assessment system, nurse tutors were now responsible for conducting assessments and this ended the practice of matrons and doctors conducting oral examinations. The new method of clinical assessment placed the student's clinical learning on a more formal footing and gave registered nurses explicit responsibility for the assessment and, by implication, the training of students.[18] In its operation, the ward sister or a senior staff nurse was required to assess the individual student's performance over a period of time, usually six weeks, and to certify her as proficient. This required the establishment of a new professional relationship between student nurses and registered nurses, a relationship that was based on the former's explicit education and training needs and the latter's implied role as a professional gatekeeper.

In 1989 a new European directive, Directive 89/595/EEC, defined the balance that should be achieved between theoretical and clinical instruction:

> The theoretical instruction … shall be balanced and coordinated with clinical instruction … in such a way that the knowledge and experience … may be

acquired in an adequate manner. The length of the theoretical instruction shall amount to no less than one-third and that of the clinical instruction to no less than one-half of the minimum length of training.[19]

The Irish Government adopted Directive 89/595/EEC in October 1991 and, in response to the Directive, the Nursing Board published *Rules and Criteria for the Education and Training of Student Nurses* in December 1991.[20] Once operational, the new Directive required training schools to increase the duration of theoretical instruction from twenty-eight to forty weeks.

The requirements of the new Directive presented nurse tutors with an opportunity to design a new and expanded curriculum, and the Nursing Board organized a series of national seminars and workshops to assist nurse tutors in the task in hand. The extended periods of instruction provided opportunities for innovative teaching, and subjects such as research methods, communication skills and health policy were afforded greater prominence in the curriculum.[21] However, given that the nurse's primary role remained that of hospital nurse, instruction continued to place emphasis on the development of knowledge and skills for that role.

Where nurse tutors were presented with new opportunities to develop innovative teaching, hospital matrons were presented with a new challenge of meeting the staffing shortfall that resulted from students being unavailable for nursing service for an additional fourteen weeks. Providing students with forty weeks of block instruction and a range of external specialist clinical placements required a judicious balancing of duty rosters in order to maintain staffing levels in the hospital.[22]

The various European directives on nursing represented the most significant development in curriculum policy since the establishment of the General Nursing Council for Ireland in 1920. Their significance was not merely in their impact on curriculum structures, but in the fact that they transgressed the hospital's prerogative in the way that it organized the training of its nurses. No longer could the hospital provide a training largely on its own terms, but it had to provide training in compliance with the student's explicit statutory requirements and entitlements.[23]

While the European directives had an impact on the curriculum structure, their impact on staff planning in the training hospitals was to have more far-reaching consequences for the system of apprenticeship nurse training in Ireland. Where the first directives of 1977 rendered the nurse training system as a much less cost-effective means of securing trained nurses, Directive 89/595/EEC placed the future viability of the entire system in question.

Recruitment and selection

While the European directives brought considerable change in the structure and content of instruction, many of the features of the apprenticeship system remained. In the 1980s, the profile of the recruit to nursing had changed little since the 1960s; recruits from a rural background continued to be strongly represented and there were few men and even fewer applicants from overseas.[24] By 1990, recruitment continued to focus almost exclusively on school leavers, despite demographic patterns indicating greater participation of married women in the labour market.[25] The typical recruit was a young woman of between seventeen and nineteen years, with a good standard of secondary education and from a middle-class and/or farming rural background.[26] The personality characteristics of the women entering nursing were assessed as being 'more enthusiastic, cheerful, talkative, happy-go-lucky, quick and alert than the general population norms'.[27]

Recruitment and selection remained the prerogative of the individual hospital or health board. Recruitment patterns reflected the student's role as worker, with employers operating a constant replacement system, whereby new recruits replaced each cohort exiting the training programme.[28] Selection was made on the basis of an interview. Places in training schools were keenly contested; most candidates made separate and multiple applications in order to secure a place.[29] This process represented an economic burden for individual applicants and the screening and selection process was labour intensive for the recruiting institutions. The high levels of wastage at the point of initial recruitment and at the selection interview stage suggested that the system was inefficient and expensive.[30]

On the basis of a recommendation of the Working Party on General Nursing and acting in accordance with the provisions of the Nurses Act of 1985, the Nursing Board established a Central Applications Bureau (CAB) in 1986.[31] The CAB was established as a way of ensuring consistency and uniformity in the recruitment and selection of nurses and by 1987 the Board had put in place the necessary administrative structures, including a liaison mechanism with the Central Applications Office (CAO).[32] However, even as the new structures were being established, strong opposition was emerging from a number of the voluntary hospitals and health boards on the grounds that the proposed CAB threatened their independence in selecting staff. Among the strongest opponents were the three principal denominational hospitals in Dublin, the Catholic Mater Misericordiae and St Vincent's hospitals and the Protestant Adelaide Hospital, and each institution took its concerns directly to the Minister for Health Dr Rory O'Hanlon.[33] While the Minister supported in principle the establishment of the CAB, he also upheld the right of independent institutions to select their own trainee nurses.[34] In the face of such strong opposition, the Nursing Board was forced to abandon the new central applications scheme in July 1987.[35] The Board had not reckoned on the influence and the determination of powerful vested interests. Despite its chastening experience, the Nursing Board continued to promote the idea of a centralized recruitment and selection system.[36]

Pedagogy

For most student nurses in 1980, the school of nursing was a place of sanctuary from the demands of a busy hospital. A principal nurse tutor managed the nursing school and a growing number of nurse tutors gave the instruction.[37] In the clinical setting, the student nurse's experience was of work rather than learning;

she routinely undertook non-nursing duties and there was a lack of clinical teaching.[38] In 1980, the Working Party on General Nursing had expressed concern at a dissonance between nurse tutors' teaching and the reality of clinical practice, noting that teachers were becoming 'isolated and remote from the main areas of nursing activities'.[39] Despite the abiding concern to achieve closer links between the nurse tutor and clinical practice, evidence from successive formal inspections of schools of nursing by the Nursing Board indicated that the situation had not improved.[40] Aside from the additional teaching required under the European directives, many nurse tutors had extended their role into continuing education and into nursing development projects. Many became increasingly de-skilled as clinicians and some felt out of touch with new developments and uneasy in the clinical area.[41] By the early 1990s, it was increasingly apparent that many nurse tutors had all but abandoned their clinical teaching role, thereby limiting the range of learning opportunities available to students and adversely affecting the overall quality of students' clinical learning.

Prevailing paradigms of curriculum and instruction within general education influenced nursing education. The behavioural-objectives model was especially prevalent in Irish schools of nursing, where it was not unusual to find copious lists of objectives relating to every possible aspect of student learning.[42] The model provided nurse tutors with the pedagogical means of ensuring that theoretical and clinical instruction could be carefully prescribed and the outcomes measured. Notwithstanding the preponderance of learning objectives, in the relatively small class sizes that obtained in the schools of nursing, nurse tutors could experiment with and develop student-centred pedagogies.[43] As Cowman wrote, these pedagogies, with their implicit humanistic values, were presented to students within the behavioural-objectives framework, and in their teaching content, many nurse tutors were espousing a humanistic philosophy as the basis for clinical nursing.[44] The (abridged) ideas of writers like Abraham Maslow and Carl Rogers were frequently invoked in the classroom, and the lexicon of nursing content contained expressions like 'individualized care', 'patient-centred care' and 'holistic care'. Humanism emerged in the curriculum through the influence of trends in international nursing literature and was promoted through the educational preparation of nurse tutors at University College Dublin in the 1980s. Andragogical theory was a particular version of humanism to which many nurse tutors subscribed; while undergoing assessments of their teaching skills, it was *de rigueur* for nurse tutors to prepare a student-centred lesson plan. Notwithstanding these efforts at 'progressive' teaching, in a paradoxical way, the behavioural-objectives model prevailed, and didactic teaching strategies remained the dominant pedagogical medium in the classroom.[45]

Research conducted in Ireland and the United Kingdom in the 1980s indicated that the curriculum was the principal medium through which the process of professional socialization of the nurse took place.[46] While not normally explicit, underlying social processes occurring in and through the curriculum were powerful in shaping the student's training experiences and her subsequent ability and scope as a trained nurse.[47] The student's professional socialization was achieved through the messages that she received concerning her professional role and aspects of her training. Through the curriculum, she was given to understand that she was first and foremost a worker who was expected to be passive, compliant, and to willingly serve.[48] This work ethic was transmitted in the form of priorities and work routines and in the fact that the student nurse was required to assume worker responsibilities.[49] In her clinical placements, she quickly learned the ethic of 'getting the work done', and her passive role in the delivery of care was reinforced through an emphasis on the performance of tasks and through the hierarchical structure of the ward.[50] Tasks typically involved two-hourly toilet, four-hourly observations, four-hourly reflochecks, two-hourly vital signs, oral care, and 'settling the patients'.[51] Student nurses realized that knowing the ward routine was all that was needed to 'get by' and they could derive comfort from the certainty of this routine.[52]

Through a highly structured curriculum with rigid timetabling and an emphasis on subject separateness and knowledge transmission, the student could experience the curriculum as a 'quiescent recipient'.[53] The lack of connectedness between subjects meant that students could sense a failure to relate classroom knowledge to their clinical experience.[54]

Proposals for reform

The weaknesses of the system of nurse training were held to reside principally in the inherent weakness of the model of apprenticeship training.[55] Apprenticeship training placed the student nurse in an ambiguous role of worker and learner and much of her clinical experiences had little to do with the development of clinical skills.[56] The curriculum was considered to be disjointed and with little thought given to the rationale for certain clinical placements other than their ability to address the needs of hospital nursing service. These dysfunctions of apprenticeship training led to proposals for reform that included calls for a university degree in nursing.

As early as 1973, there was the prospect of an entry-level baccalaureate degree in nursing, when the Governing Body of University College Galway (UCG) gave approval in principle to the establishment of such a programme.[57] However, this programme did not commence and it would be a further two decades before UCG would again feature in initiatives to establish academic recognition for basic nurse training. In 1980, with the exception of the Nurse Tutors' Diploma at University College Dublin, the diploma courses for registered nurses offered by the Royal College of Surgeons in Ireland, and courses in hospital administration offered by some regional technical colleges and colleges of commerce, links between nursing and higher education were tenuous and few.[58] Nursing had not been a priority for the higher education sector. However, many higher education institutions would come to see involvement in nurse training as a means of increasing their technical-vocational remit. While finance and accommodation were obstacles to the entry of nursing into higher education, the principal obstacle remained the central role that the student nurse played in the delivery of hospital nursing services.

In the years between 1980 and 1992, the Nursing Board received a total of six submissions from universities and health boards, each proposing a new academic programme of pre-registration education and training.[59] Reflecting the recommendations of the Working Party on General Nursing, each submission contained a proposal for a common core model of training, and at least two proposed a degree in nursing. However, none of these proposals were implemented.

In the 1990s, recognizing the difficulties that apprenticeship training presented for student learning, most commentators on nursing were in favour of placing nurse training within an academic framework. Some nursing leaders were divided on the requirement for graduate education at the point of registration, and others disagreed as to the form that a reformed system of training should take. Disagreement centred on the sort of educational model that should replace the apprenticeship model. In 1990, Geraldine McCarthy, a senior nurse manager at Dublin's Beaumont Hospital, proposed a bachelor of nursing degree to be located in universities and colleges of higher education under the auspices of the Department of Education.[60] The proposed degree would prepare a generalist nurse and nursing students could receive interdisciplinary instruction in foundation science subjects from other university faculties. McCarthy argued that nursing students needed and deserved a broad education:

> I personally deplore any attempt to narrow the concept of nurse education in academia into a monotechnic structure in which nursing students are taught only by nurses as a replication or extension of the traditional system.[61]

McCarthy acknowledged that the introduction of the proposed degree would be constrained by factors such as funding and opposition from within and from outside the profession, and she also raised the question as to whether universities needed or wanted nursing.[62]

Seamus Cowman, an education officer at the Nursing Board, questioned the proposal concerning the preparation of a generalist nurse with its implied abandoning of the psychiatric, mental handicap and paediatric nursing branches, and he called for an analysis of the apprenticeship system before its replacement by any alternative model.[63] He also cautioned that the effort needed in preparing the health service workforce for the change to an alternative system of training should not be underestimated.

With the weight of international opinion strongly in favour of ending the student nurse's dual role of worker and student, it is unsurprising that the Nursing Board should adopt this same position. Arising out of the recommendations of the Report of the Working Party on General Nursing in 1980 and following developments in the United Kingdom that saw the attainment of academic recognition for basic nurse training, the Nursing Board took a policy decision that basic nurse training in Ireland should be moved from the hospital into higher education.[64] The Board argued that such a move would improve the scope and quality of education, rationalize the system of training, contain costs and improve patient care through the procurement of a highly trained and stable workforce. While the

Board was mindful of the enormous staffing implications that the proposed move would entail, it nevertheless foresaw the attainment of full student status for nursing students as a desirable goal. In 1987, the Board's President Sr Columba McNamara declared:

> It is imperative that we in Ireland move now on third level education ... as well as providing for the needs of the Health Services, we must also consider the needs of the young people for whom we are providing the education.[65]

The Nursing Board moved on its policy position in February 1989 when it decided that a review of pre- and post-registration nursing education was warranted; in September 1990, it established a committee to undertake the review.[66] The Review Committee consisted of twenty-one members, twelve of whom were Board representatives, with the remaining nine members representing health boards, voluntary hospitals, the Higher Education Authority, and the National Council for Educational Awards. The Review Committee was remitted to conduct an analysis of the strengths and weaknesses of the system of nurse training, and make proposals regarding training, examinations and post-registration training.

In the following year, the Review Committee published an Interim Report.[67] The report presented an analysis of the system of pre-registration education and training, in the light of labour force and staffing issues, demographic trends and epidemiological patterns, and national and international health policies. On the basis of research that demonstrated the inherent shortcomings of apprenticeship training and mindful of demographic and illness patterns and national health policy, the Review Committee concluded that the system of nurse training in Ireland needed reform. The case for reform was based on a number of 'key factors'. These were the shifting policies towards health promotion and community health, significant demographic trends and epidemiological patterns, the requirement for nursing service to be efficient and cost effective, and the need to rationalize and strengthen the process of nursing education to accord with European and international developments.

A particular concern of the Review Committee was the capacity of nurse training to develop and support nursing service in accordance with future health needs, especially in light of the changing definitions of health and healthcare. It presented three alternative models of nurse training: the existing 'specialist' model, a 'generalist' model, and a 'common core' model with specialist elements, and it pointed out that the generalist and common core models could be implemented at either diploma or degree level. The Review Committee concluded its report with a list of key issues for discussion that included the formation of structures for a centralized system of applications to nursing, academic recognition for nursing qualifications, and the status of future students of nursing. In citing the common core model as a key issue for future discussion, the Review Committee was implicitly upholding the earlier recommendation of the Working Party on General Nursing by offering the common core model as its preferred option.

Following the publication of the Interim Report, the Nursing Board invited submissions from interested parties, and through a series of regional seminars, it facilitated a process of nationwide consultation with nurses. This process led to the publication of the Nursing Board's report, entitled *The Future of Nurse Education and Training in Ireland*, in 1994.[68] In the report, the Board again highlighted deficiencies in the apprenticeship system of nurse training, which it attributed to 'a lack of student nurses' preparedness for certain duties, a lack of clinical teaching and an emphasis on work rather than learning'. Building on the findings of the Interim Report, the new report reprised the factors that supported the need for change, citing the dysfunctional aspects of the student's dual status as worker and learner, the changing trends in healthcare, and a recruitment policy that was failing to take account of staff planning.

The Future of Nurse Education and Training in Ireland contained twenty-eight recommendations on the organizational, educational and economic issues concerning the future of nursing in Ireland. The Board recommended the establishment of a central applications system, the withdrawal of the student's requirement to provide nursing service, and full student status for students of nursing. It called for the establishment of links with higher education for the purpose of educational validation and accreditation of nursing programmes, but did not propose the wholesale entry of nursing into the higher education sector. Instead, the Board envisaged a rationalization of existing schools of nursing and midwifery, leading to the establishment of colleges of nursing and midwifery. The report did not specify the level of the academic award to be made at the point of registration.

As hinted at in the Interim Report, the Nursing Board's preferred framework for pre-registration education and training was the common core model, a model that was similar to the United Kingdom Central Council's 'Project 2000', an entry-level diploma model. However, the common core model was not the preferred choice of the Department of Health, which communicated its opposition to the Board at the time.[69] The Department's opposition stemmed partly from a concern that the model might adversely affect recruitment to the specialist branches, such as learning disabilities and mental health. The President of the Nursing Board Ita O'Dwyer expressed confidence that any differences of view with the Department of Health could be addressed in and through consultation and experimentation with new models of education and training.[70]

The Minister for Health Brendan Howlin accepted the broad thrust of *The Future of Nurse Education and Training in Ireland*. As part of the Government's health strategy, he saw the necessity to 'align the regime for nursing education more closely with the demands of the modern day health service'.[71] The Minister envisaged an overhaul of nurse training, which would include active input from third-level colleges of education and formal accreditation of educational and training achievements. In line with the Government's commitment to community care, the Minister also envisaged changes in the curriculum, including the allocation of more time for community placements. Representing 'the single most significant investment in nursing education in recent decades', the Minister gave notice that the process of change would begin in 1994 and would be implemented as speedily as possible.[72]

The Galway Model and academic recognition

The impetus for change, begun in 1991 with the Review Committee's Interim Report, was sustained by the publication of *The Future of Nurse Education and Training in Ireland* in 1994, by the Minister for Health's pronouncements, and by a strong desire for change within the profession. Anticipation that change was inevitable was heightened by the fact that the UKCC's 'Project 2000' pre-registration diploma programme had been recently introduced in Northern Ireland.[73] All that remained for the change to occur was the provision of the necessary government funding for one or more initiatives.

While the profession anticipated change in 1994, it had not anticipated the source, direction or rapidity of the change. On the same day that the Minister for Health formally received *The Future of Nurse Education and Training in Ireland* report, he announced the introduction of a pilot scheme for a diploma in nursing at UCG.[74] Conjointly prepared by UCG and the Western Health Board, the scheme had been submitted for approval to the Department of Health and to the Nursing Board. The scheme was prepared in parallel with, but independent of, the Nursing Board's consultative process that led to the publication of *The Future of Nurse Education and Training in Ireland*.

UCG and the Western Health Board had begun collaborating in the area of nursing education as early as 1980. At that time, the college had obtained approval in principle from the Nursing Board for a degree in nursing.[75] In 1991, UCG and the Western Health Board established a Joint Nurse Education Working Party to examine nurse training requirements in the light of European Directive 89/595/EEC and the university's accreditation requirements. The Joint Nurse Education Working Party recommended a rolling four-year degree programme with an exit option at diploma level, and this proposal was approved by the college authorities and was entered into the UCG Calendar for the academic session 1994–1995. The Joint Nurse Education Working Party also recommended the establishment of a Department of Nursing Studies at UCG, to be headed by 'an academic of some standing in the field of nursing'.[76]

The Galway pilot scheme awarded a Diploma in Nursing Studies at the point of registration after three years, and students could opt to pursue an additional academic year of studies leading to the award of a degree in nursing. The scheme conferred full student status on the student nurse and made her supernumerary to service for all but a fourteen-week period of the three-year programme. For the first time in Ireland, a link was established between a health authority and a university for the purpose of academic accreditation of a basic nurse training programme. The so-called 'Galway Model' aimed to build on existing programmes of pre-registration training, enhancing rather than totally changing the traditional system.[77] The programme of study complied with the requirements for registration with the Nursing Board and it incorporated long periods of clinical instruction, thereby maintaining the clinical practice ethic, which valued a clinically based education and training.[78] Since the Western Health Board already employed the nurse tutors who would teach the main elements of the programme, the only significant additional costs were related to the teaching of biological and social sciences. Recruitment of students was based on the projected numbers required for the services.[79]

Indicating that the Galway pilot scheme was the beginning of a major overhaul of the system of nurse training in Ireland, the Minister for Health presided over the official launch of the scheme on 22 September 1994.[80] Having approved the scheme on a pilot basis, the Nursing Board welcomed the initiative as the foundation for the future development of nurse training in Ireland.[81] The Board's Chief Executive Officer Eugene Donoghue declared that the scheme was 'a significant and momentous step in the education and training of student nurses'.[82]

In approving the Galway scheme, the Nursing Board was following the Department of Health's policy position, which supported academic recognition in principle, and it congratulated the Minister for 'taking determined action' in line with the recommendations contained in *The Future of Nurse Education and Training in Ireland*. However, the scheme and the manner of its introduction were at variance with one of the fundamental elements of the Board's own policy position. A key recommendation contained in the *The Future of Nurse Education and Training in Ireland* was the common core model as the preferred educational framework. This recommendation was not adopted.[83] Instead, the Galway scheme retained the specialist model of training and, with it, the distinction between the specialist branches of nursing at the point of entry to nurse training. The Nursing Board had previously adjudged the specialist model to be not rational, not economic, and not in the interests of the employer or the client of nursing service. The Galway Model appeared to run counter to the wishes of the Board and those of the profession at that time. Nevertheless, the Galway initiative could not have been taken to the point of final validation and approval without the assent and the necessary consultation between UCG, the Western Health Board and the Nursing Board.[84]

Despite its view that a common core model was the 'the best option', the Nursing Board acknowledged that the Galway scheme set out the broad direction in which nurse training could expect to develop.[85] While the Galway scheme was ostensibly launched on a pilot basis, the Department of Health declared that the scheme was the model to which all other institutions of higher education should subscribe. Many institutions felt wrong-footed and at a strategic disadvantage. This was especially true of those institutions that had previously and independently developed pre-registration nursing diploma or degree programmes. Nevertheless, while most resented an externally imposed educational framework, they were keen to commence the diploma programme based on the Galway Model at the earliest opportunity. Furthermore, the Irish Nurses' Organisation declared that the profession would not countenance a two-tier system of training, leading to a two-tier grade of nurse.[86]

In the ensuing three years, the other principal universities and institutions of higher education, in partnership with the voluntary hospitals and health boards, introduced the new registration-diploma course. By 1998, all of the general nurse training schools were operating the Galway Model and recruitment to the hospital apprenticeship-training programme had ceased.

In the period between 1995 and 1998, the Department of Health took an active role in directing the transition to the new diploma programme, adopting a directive and prescriptive approach and requiring educational and healthcare institutions to develop and implement the Galway Model in conformity to a highly prescribed standard.[87] The Department set out precise directives on how the partnership between the health services and the higher education sector should proceed and on how the curriculum should be developed and operated.[88] This close engagement with curriculum policy on the part of the Department was not the result of any ideological position concerning education, but was related to the control of costs connected with the running of the programme. However, by the end of the 1990s when the new programme had become consolidated nationally, the Department assumed a less hands-on approach and returned decisions concerning the minutiae of curriculum design to the curriculum planners. Aside from the tensions that accompanied the tight control maintained by the Department of Health in the transitional period, a noteworthy feature of the change process was the spirit of partnership that attended the project, and this ensured a smooth transition of nurse training from the hospital to the academy.[89]

At around the time when the Galway scheme commenced, a number of degree courses for registered nurses had been instituted, including a modular part-time degree of Bachelor of Nursing Studies for registered nurses at University College Dublin, which commenced in 1992. This and similar courses were popular and it was clear that many nurses wished to advance their professional education and training to degree level.

Conclusions

Up to 1980, international reports on nursing were calling into question the system of apprenticeship nurse training, and its ethos of work-based learning had come under increasing and sustained scrutiny.[90] In the 1980s, a substantial body of empirical research pointed to the dysfunctional aspects of apprenticeship training, which were related to the conflict between the student nurse's dual role as hospital worker and learner. Most incontrovertible was the evidence that the quality of learning was severely compromised by the incongruous status of the student nurse and there was increasing concern that the system of training ill prepared the student for the nursing role envisaged in the changing health services. Furthermore, untrained student nurses were providing coalface care to a population of patients that, following the rationalization of hospital services in the 1980s, tended to have higher levels of dependency.[91] This situation was also difficult to sustain in a milieu of growing consumerism and the need for greater professional accountability.[92]

In a health service that was highly labour intensive, the system of apprenticeship training provided a ready and a relatively inexpensive supply of hospital workers. As long as the nurse in training provided this ready and inexpensive labour, then economic policy would dictate that she should remain as a hospital employee. Were the student nurse to become economically inefficient, then the apprenticeship system might be relinquished; this eventuality was brought closer when European directives on the training of nurses were implemented in 1979 and again in 1991. Through the requirements for additional theoretical and clinical instruction, the European directives greatly reduced the student nurse's availability for work in the service of the employer. The directives also challenged the tight control that individual hospitals had in the training of nurses; the nurse's training was to be conducted on the basis of her explicit learning requirements, which were on a new statutory footing. Economic and educational imperatives were operating to bring about change.

The debate about the future of nurse training in Ireland was ongoing and had not been fully exhausted when the Galway diploma model of training was introduced on an unsuspecting profession. While the Government accepted the recommendations of *The Future of Nurse Education and Training in Ireland*, it was not prepared to permit a common point of entry to nursing or to permit the wholesale exodus of nurse training to the higher education sector. In consequence, the Galway Model was introduced in September 1994 as the only acceptable scheme to replace the apprenticeship system of training. The Galway Model was acceptable because it retained the various branches of nursing, and it maintained the student's close association with the training hospital. Furthermore, it was submitted for approval through the auspices of a health service agency and not through a higher education institution alone. In this way, nurse training remained largely under the jurisdiction of the health services. Working in the hospitals' favour was the evidence suggesting that the high levels of recruitment to nursing would be maintained if not enhanced with the advent of academic recognition. The arrangements for funding the programme also made it acceptable.

While pragmatic and fiscal considerations were the basis of the decision to end the apprenticeship system of nurse training in 1994, for many years previously the nursing profession in Ireland had demanded change, ostensibly on educational grounds. However, the procurement of academic recognition for the basic nursing qualification represented nursing's strategy at establishing greater professional status and occupational enhancement.[93] By locating itself in higher education, nursing was making a significant statement about its status as a professional discipline. In its development, nursing had, for better or worse, been closely allied to the medical profession as an ancillary 'paramedical' occupation.[94] In that position, nursing's relationship with medicine was implicitly that of a lesser partner. In its new position in higher education, nursing was redefining its professional relationships and it was declaring its professional identity and its occupational autonomy. Nursing was not merely attempting to redefine its relationship with medicine, but it was also attempting to create its own educational sphere, within which its own philosophies could be articulated.[95]

9 Conclusions

Reform has been the major theme of this book. In Ireland, modern nursing emerged as the result of a process of nursing reform, and the system of hospital apprenticeship nurse training was an integral part of that reform. The training system was itself the subject of gradual reform throughout its 115 years as a social practice, and its ending in the 1990s was also part of the process of educational reform experienced by nursing in Ireland and in the United Kingdom in the period.

Relationships

The reform of nursing was a significant social movement in Ireland in the late nineteenth century, and it represented part of the wider trend in women's labour patterns in the period. The movement was less an example of an unexpected revolution and more the result of the convergence of interrelated social developments and trends occurring in the wake of the Industrial Revolution. The advent of the modern nurse was a logical consequence of the confluence of scientific progress, militarism, changed thinking on the role of women as workers, the suffragist movement, and the women's education movement. The establishment of nursing as a middle-class secular-professional social practice was thus part of a wider process of social change in the nineteenth century and involving women and their role in society.

Nursing reform removed lower-class women from hospital nursing, replacing them with young middle-class women, drawn from a 'better class of person'. Provided with instruction in the theory and practice of sick nursing, the reformed nurse was made responsible for nursing care and hospital sanitation. The first leaders of modern nursing in Ireland were gentlewomen of Anglo-Irish, English or Scottish parentage and were the daughters of professionals, including medical men and military officers. While some probationers were drawn from a similar social background, the ranks of probationers were mostly rural-provincial young women; a ready supply of the daughters of small farmers and artisans provided the recruits to nursing throughout the twentieth century. While nursing reform altered the class basis of nursing, their lower-middle-class social background, their gender and the nature of their work meant that nurses did not enjoy the same social or professional status as the members of equivalent professional disciplines, such as teaching. Furthermore, the system of apprenticeship training meant that nursing remained outside the learned professions.

Like the teaching profession, modern nursing became a predominantly female domain activity and, along with teaching, it presented middle-class women with a way of entering paid professional work at a time when there were few opportunities for women to enter the public sphere. Nursing contained many parallels with the teaching profession, and many of the social factors operating in the late Victorian period, such as scientific progress and women's suffrage, converged to bring about the emergence of the professional teacher and the professional nurse. As both professions developed, their histories continued to exhibit parallels. Nursing and teaching were predominantly women's professions whose direction and management were controlled by men and/or by a male worldview; men teachers became the powerbrokers within teaching, while male doctors became powerbrokers of nursing. While nursing remained an essentially female profession, it developed and evolved in such a way that it was top-down managed in a manner similar to a male profession. For example, hierarchical structures in the hospital's nursing department established relationships of authority that mirrored male hierarchical systems such as the military; the uniform inspection in nursing had an obvious parallel in the military.[1]

While the nurse–doctor dyad was a significant social relationship in the clinical arena, the relationship of nursing to medicine was an expression of the wider gender relationship that determined women's experiences in education and in the workplace. The experiences of nurses in training were intimately bound up with this broader gender relationship, and the relationship determined the way that nurse training evolved, both at the broader policy level and at the micro level of the curriculum.

In the nineteenth century, with its growing involvement in medical relief and medical training, hospital medicine based on empirical science became the dominant model of healthcare in Ireland. The project of scientific medicine succeeded in achieving its dominant position in the voluntary hospital and in the wider community, partly because of the success of the project of nursing reform, which provided a trained nurse who could meet the needs of the medical man and the sick patient. While hospital scientific medicine depended on the reformed hospital nurse, the new discipline of nursing came to depend on scientific medicine for its *raison d'être*. In this way, medicine and nursing evolved in a relationship of interdependence.

However, with its monopoly position over diagnosis and prescription, medicine was the dominant partner in the relationship. This dominance was also a function of the gender dominance of men over women and the class difference between doctors and nurses. Through nursing reform, nursing tied itself to the medical profession and to medical knowledge in a way that determined the status of the nurse as a worker in a position ancillary to medicine.[2] In the process, the medical profession tended to be the principal powerbroker of the nursing profession, as the latter interacted with officialdom.

While the medical profession continued to be the principal powerbroker of nursing, new powerbrokers emerged in the twentieth century, including the Hierarchy of the Catholic Church and the Civil Service. Nevertheless, nursing leaders were able to negotiate and moderate the influence of its external powerbrokers in ways that brought nursing forward towards the achievement of its own desired goals.

Where many nursing leaders succeeded in advancing the development of nursing towards full professional status, others were complicit in retarding its development. This was especially so in the way that some nursing leaders propagated idealized images of the nurse. In professional discourse, there was type and there was stereotype, and there was a fairly rigid conformity to the archetypal 'good nurse' image, with its associations with womanhood, Christian devotion, and loyalty to the institution and to the medical profession.[3] In its failure to challenge the stereotype, some nursing leaders inadvertently maintained for the nurse the status of the trained worker, as opposed to that of the learned professional. Professional identity and status were formed in a way that accorded with these idealized images. Moreover, the nursing profession was also complicit in sustaining the dependent relationship with medicine, in the way that it relied upon the medical profession to teach and assess its nurses in training.

Just as hospital scientific medicine had come to represent the dominant paradigm of medical care, hospital nursing became the dominant paradigm of sick nursing. In this way, the hospital was the locus of nurse training, and hospital nursing was the focus of the training experience. Despite efforts by successive governments since the 1940s to promote a social model of healthcare, the role of the hospital nurse continued to be the dominant role that the nurse performed and this role represented the principal justification for the curriculum.

The system of hospital apprenticeship training in Ireland functioned to train a competent and caring worker to provide sick nursing in the hospital wards, and the trainee's curricular experiences were also aimed at socializing her into her chosen profession, its ideals and its value systems. Through explicit and implicit messages contained in the content of instruction, the student nurse learned about her position in the hospital structure, and about her relationships with her employer, her superiors, the doctor and the patient. Through the gestalt of her experiences in block, on the wards and in the nurses' home, she received messages about what was to be valued in nursing. She learned the ideals of good nursing and the values of hard work, obedience to authority, loyalty to the training hospital, accurate reporting, attention to detail in nursing work, attentiveness to the patient's needs, and kindness to the patient. Through instruction and examinations, she also learned the value of medical knowledge. The student nurse was also presented with experiences that demanded deference to authority and conformity to strict rules that governed her work, her studies and her leisure.

Change

Social history provides indicators that predicted change and development in nursing in Ireland. New social relationships between the rich and the poor following the Industrial Revolution, the gendered division of labour, and the development of scientific medicine each predicted the reform of nursing in the nineteenth century. In the early twentieth century, predictors of change in nursing included women's suffrage, and the experiences of a new State in its transition from an agrarian to an industrial society. The attainment of professional regulation was the most significant event in the development of modern nursing and it paralleled the attainment of women's suffrage. Predictors of change in the late twentieth century included the communications revolution that began with television in the 1960s, new understanding of the concept of 'profession', the removal of the marriage bar on women in the civil and public services, prevailing economic circumstances, educational policy more generally, and the changing role of the universities.

The development of modern nursing in Ireland was intimately bound up with the wider developments occurring in Irish society. The transition in social and political power and influence, which occurred in the period between the late nineteenth century and the middle of the twentieth century, brought fundamental changes in Irish public life.[4] In the late nineteenth century, a liberal Anglo-Irish Protestant intelligentsia was the driving force behind the social reform movement that included nursing and sanitary reform. By the middle of the twentieth century, the Protestant tradition of philanthropy and social reform was less influential in macro social policy. Catholics had replaced Protestants in many public institutions and in the Civil Service, and social policy came under the influence of a more conservative Catholic-nationalist worldview. Since the leaders of nursing and the powerbrokers behind them were drawn from the same respective Protestant and Catholic constituencies that, in their turn, dominated Irish public life, nursing also witnessed a transition in the derivation of its values and its power and influence. The transition was particularly relevant in the way that the nurse was portrayed in public discourses; the nineteenth-century image of lady nursing as 'that highest walk of woman's work' was gradually replaced with an image that invoked vocation and self-denial, Catholic devotion to duty, and the 'good practical nurse'.[5] The development of nursing in Ireland was also influenced by the prevailing state of the economy, which affected the state of the health services, and by interest groups, most especially the public voluntary hospitals, the medical profession, and the Roman Catholic hierarchy.

In popular discourse, the quality of nurse training in Ireland was frequently declared to be among the best in the world. However, hospital apprenticeship training in Ireland was, in some respects, of dubious quality. Student nurses were recruited principally as workers and their training was aimed at the acquisition of work-related skills. Nurse training was conducted in a way that fostered subservience to authority and compliance with rules that appeared more often concerned with personal behaviour than with the development of the professional role.

From the 1950s onwards, the system of apprenticeship nurse training became the subject of professional debate in Ireland. While some commentators evaluated the system in a positive light, doubts were raised about the validity of a training system that was conducted in institutions that were not educational in nature, and the failure to render the nursing school independent of the hospital was seen as a significant factor in retarding the development of nurse training. In the 1980s, beginning with the Report of the Working Party on General Nursing, the system came under sustained scrutiny. Concerns were raised about the appropriateness of the apprenticeship system for the training of nurses, with the principal concern resting on the conflict inherent in the nurse's dual role as employee and learner. The system was questioned on the grounds that it was failing to meet the training needs of nurses for their new roles in healthcare. Epidemiological trends in altered health, advances in science, and health policy were invoked to demonstrate the limited perspective that hospital apprenticeship training offered. While the system contained a clinical practice ethic that valued clinical-based training, the student's pre-eminent responsibilities to her employer were increasingly rendering her learning as a subordinate activity. In the process, her skills were limited to her need to function as a proficient nurse in her training hospital.

When new European directives on the training of nurses were implemented in 1979 and again in 1991, the system became unsustainable, principally on economic grounds. Economic considerations also determined the direction that nurse training took as it made the move from the hospital to the academy. Academic recognition was achieved with a partial integration of nurse training into the academy. Despite the desire on the part of the nursing profession to disconnect professional training from nursing service, the Government maintained an employer-led system of training by its promotion of the Galway Model of diploma-level training.

Postscript

Following a period of industrial unrest related to pay, promotional opportunities and related matters, a Commission on Nursing was established in March 1997.[6] The Commission on Nursing examined a broad range of issues related to nursing and midwifery in Ireland, such as the evolving role of nurses and midwives, promotional opportunities, the requirements placed on nurses both in training and in delivery of service, and the training and educational requirements of nurses. The Commission presented nursing in Ireland with an opportunity to synthesize the views of Irish nurses and to formulate these into recommendations, which would be the source of appropriate policies.[7] The Commission provided the impetus for the establishment of a degree programme for pre-registration training.[8]

In presenting its final report, entitled *A Blueprint for the Future*, in the autumn of 1998, the Commission aimed to 'provide a secure basis for the further professional development of nursing in the context of anticipated changes in health services, their organization and delivery'.[9] The Commission made recommendations on a wide range of issues pertaining to nursing and midwifery, including recommendations on the educational preparation for the profession in Ireland. The new registration-diploma Galway Model, introduced in 1994, was adjudged to have failed to offer the student nurse the full benefits of a third-level education. The Commission cited international trends towards degree-level education for nurses in Australia, New Zealand, Canada and the United States. It called for the full integration of pre-registration training into third-level institutes of higher education, and it recommended that the future framework for the pre-registration education be based on a four-year degree programme. The Commission specified the year 2002 as the start-up date for the commencement of the proposed new programme.

The Government accepted the recommendations of the Commission on Nursing, and it provided the necessary funding to permit the establishment of new schools of nursing in the universities and in a number of institutes of technology. In September 2002, the first cohort of undergraduate nursing students entered the new programme and nurse training became fully integrated into higher education.

Notes

1 Charity, medical relief and precursors of the modern nurse

1 Summers, 1989a, pp. 31–7.
2 MacLurg Jensen, 1959, p. 93.
3 Daly, 1981.
4 Cited in Helmstadter, 2003, pp. 2–30.
5 Summers, 1989a, p. 32.
6 Knibiehler, 1993, pp. 325–68.
7 Scott, 1993, pp. 399–426.
8 Ibid., pp. 401–2. Scott writes that the discourse surrounding women as workers drew on medical, scientific, political and moral opinion concerning the role of women and was presented in terms of the separation of the home from the workplace and the gender division of labour. Scott points out that commentators ignored the fact that most women workers were young and single, implying that they would not have the sort of domestic responsibilities ascribed to them.
9 Ibid., p. 426.
10 As an explanatory model, the 'separate spheres' theory serves as a framework for discussing the experiences of women in the post-Industrial Revolution period. However, a number of writers have challenged the validity of the separate spheres model. See Luddy, 1995, p. 2. On the basis of extant critiques and doubts concerning the validity of the model, Simonton cautions that women's historians need to question their methodology and approach rather than accept the separate spheres model as a truism. See Simonton, 2001, pp. 35–47. In clarifying the origins of the separate spheres theory, Summers casts further doubt on its validity, proposing that the idea of separate spheres was a construction of nineteenth-century narrative introduced into popular debate, and that women did in fact participate actively in public life. See Summers, 2000, Chapter 1. Scott proposes that the 'doctrine of separate spheres' interpretation of the history of women as workers might be better referred to as the discourse that conceptualized gender as the 'natural' division of labour. See Scott, 1993, pp. 399–426. See also Vickery, 1998.
11 Slater, 1994, pp. 137–52.
12 Helmstadter, 2003, p. 4.
13 D'Antonio, 1997, pp. 16–7. See also Summers, 1989a, p. 32. This value system is often referred to as the Victorian 'cult of domesticity', which held the home to be the sanctuary of morality, a place where the poor moral condition of society at large would not be allowed to enter; the woman was held to be the guardian of this sanctuary. See, for example, Rafferty, 1996, p. 26.
14 Helmstadter, 1993a, pp. 282–319.
15 Helmstadter, 2001, pp. 127–40.
16 Ibid., p. 128.

17 Davies, 1987, pp. 111–22.
18 Ibid., p. 119.
19 Daly, 1984, p. 270.
20 Ibid.
21 Ibid., p. 276.
22 MacLurg Jenson, 1959, chapter 6.
23 Baubérot, 1993, pp. 198–212. In the case of Dublin, wealthier class is taken to denote the Anglo-Irish nobility.
24 Luddy, 1995, p. 1.
25 Helmstadter, 1993a, p. 291.
26 Luddy, 1995, p. 1.
27 Helmstadter, 2001, pp. 127 and 129.
28 Basford, 1995, pp. 25–48.
29 Summera, 1989, p. 33.
30 Nelson, 1999, pp.171–87.
31 Summers. 1989b, pp. 365–86.
32 Baly, 1987, p. 5.
33 Denny, 1997, pp. 1175–82
34 Helmstadter, 1993a, pp. 282–3.
35 Helmstadter, 2001, pp. 127–40.
36 Luddy, 1995, pp. 56–9 and 63; Luddy, 1997.
37 Luddy, 1995, p. 62.
38 Francis, 2001, pp. 169–76; Clear, 1987.
39 Nelson, 2001, chapter 2.
40 Francis, 2001, p. 172.
41 Meehan, 2003, pp. 99–107.
42 Luddy, 1999, pp. 102–17.
43 Luddy, 1995, p. 50; Nelson, 1997, pp. 6–14.
44 Helmstadter, 2001, pp. 130–1.
45 Doona, 1995, pp. 3–41.
46 Doona, 1999; Bolster, 1964.
47 Nelson, 1997, p. 8.
48 Ibid. p. 13.
49 Meehhan, 2003, p. 99.
50 Fahey, 1988, pp. 411–29.
51 Ibid., p. 415.
52 Luddy, 1999, p. 107; Nelson, 1997, p. 7.
53 Luddy, 1999, p. 115.
54 Banks, 1883.
55 O'Brien, 1988, p. 3.
56 House of Commons, hereafter cited as HC, 1838, (38), iii, 451.
57 Ibid., p. 80.
58 House, 1987, p. xii.
59 Ibid.
60 Burke, 1987, p. 20.
61 Barrington, 1987, p. 5.
62 Kelly, 1972, p. 7.
63 White, 1978, p. 7.
64 Dean and Bolton, 1980, pp. 76–101.
65 Cited in Kelly, 1972, p. 5.
66 Burke, 1987, p. 68.
67 Luddy, 1999, p. 103.
68 HC, 1854, (383), xii1., p. 63 (evidence of Alfred Power).
69 Scanlan, 1991, p. 6.

70 Burke, 1987, p. 289.
71 Ibid.
72 HC, 1863. See also Barrington, 1987, p. 8; Burke, 1987, p. 298.
73 Luddy, 1999, p. 103.
74 Daly, 1984, p. 39.
75 Ibid. p. 86.
76 Cited in Kelly, 1972, pp.43–4.
77 Cited in Burke, 1987, p. 93.
78 HC, 1854, p. 94 (evidence of Henry Price). In 1854 it was reported that the total pop-
     ulation of the South Dublin Union workhouse was 3,720.
79 Ibid., p. 103 (evidence of Dr George B. Owens).
80 Ibid., p. 14.
81 Burke, 1987, p. 262.
82 Kelly, 1972, pp. 67–8 and 126.
83 Ibid.
84 Baly, 1977, p. 40.
85 Abel-Smith, 1960, Chapter 2. Lady Twining visited the Strand Workhouse in 1853,
     while William Rathbone visited the Liverpool Workhouse Infirmary.
86 Cited in Burke, 1987, p. 263.
87 Ibid, pp. 263–4.
88 Kelly, 1972, p. 100.
89 Cited in Burke, 1987, pp. 265–6.
90 Cited by Rev. Father P. Murray, 1968, pp. 45–50.
91 Kelly, 1972, p. 107.
92 Luddy, 1999, p. 112.
93 Ibid., p. 108.
94 Ibid., pp. 103 and 106.
95 Barrington, 1987, p. 6.
96 Luddy, 1999, p. 115
97 Barrington, 1987, pp. 9 and 55.
98 For a detailed study of the development of the early district nursing services, see
     Wickham, 2005, pp. 102–21.
99 Maclurg Jenson, 1959, p. 98.
100 Baly, 1995.
101 Wickham, 2001, pp. 26–34.
102 Dean and Bolton, 1980, p. 86.
103 O'Brien, 1984, pp. 75–114; Kelly, 1999, pp. 21–39.
104 McGeachie, 1999, pp, 85–101.
105 Ibid.
106 O'Brien, 1984, p. 75; Wolstenholme, 1984, pp. 115–46.
107 McGeachie, 1999, p. 86.
108 Ibid., p. 85. See also Fleetwood, 1951.
109 McGeachie, 1999, p. 88.
110 HC, 1854, p. 98 (evidence of Dr Thomas Brady).
111 For an account of developments in medicine and surgery in the nineteenth century,
     see Fleetwood, 1951, pp. 160–80; O'Brien *et al.*, 1984, pp. 115–46.
112 HC, 1854, p. 197 (evidence of Dr William Daniel Moore).
113 Dean and Bolton, 1980, p. 86.
114 Rumsey, 1873, p. 5 (original emphasis).
115 HC, 1887a [C.0542] xxxv.1, para xiii, p. xxxvi.
116 Helmstadter, 1993b, pp. 43–47.
117 Oakley, 1993, p.41. See also Rafferty, 1993, pp. 48–60.
118 Scanlan, 1991, pp. 16–9 and 23.
119 HC, 1854, p. 19 (evidence of Dr Thomas Byrne).

120 Helmstadter, 2003, p. 7.
121 Kirkpatrick, 1924, p. 247.
122 Abel-Smith, 1960, p. 7.
123 HC, 1854, p. xxi.
124 Kirkpatrick, 1924, p. 275.
125 Preston, 1998, vol. 2 (1), pp. 91–110.
126 HC, 1854, p. 19.
127 Dublin House of Industry Hospitals, minutes, 10 August 1871, p. 10.
128 Ibid., Minutes, 21 March, 1878, pp. 295–6.
129 Helmstadter, 2003, p. 5.
130 Preston, 1998, p. 105.
131 Rafferty, 1991, p. 43. See also Baly, 1977, p. 33.
132 Ibid., p.42.
133 Summers, 1989a, p. 34.
134 Rafferty questions whether this thesis can be substantiated on the basis that little is known about the relationship between nursing practice and medical practice. See Rafferty, 1991, p. 61.
135 Helmstadter, 1997, p. 161–97.
136 HC, 1887a, p. 27 (evidence of Mr John M. Prior Kennedy).
137 Anderson, 1897, pp. 5–6 (original emphasis).
138 Nightingale, 1969, pp. 105 and 110.
139 Rafferty, 1991, p. 51.
140 Unidentified newspaper cutting, dated 29 December 1899, inserted into Board of Directors Minute Book, City of Dublin Hospital, 11 March 1879–31 December 1899. See also Preston, 1998, p. 100; Rafferty, 1991, p. 51.
141 Cited in Summers, 1989b, p. 373.

2 'Nursing arrangements'

1 Dublin Hospital Sunday Fund, hereafter cited as DHSF, 1879; House of Commons, herafter cited as HC, 1887a [C.5042] xxxv.1, para xiii, p. xxxvi.
2 Wickham, 2001, pp. 26–34.
3 Wickham, 2000, p. 2.
4 DHSF, 1875, p. 7.
5 Ibid., p. 11.
6 HC, 1854 (383), xii.1, p. 217 (evidence of Dr Dominic Corrigan).
7 DHSF, 1876, p. 10.
8 Ibid., p. 13.
9 Ibid.
10 DHSF, 1879, p. 11.
11 The Committee was variously referred to as the 'Committee on Nursing' and the 'Nursing Committee'.
12 DHSF, 1879, p. 11. The report of the nursing arrangements was presented under the five headings of Supervision of Nursing, Qualifications and Training of Nurses, Organisation of Nursing, Wages, Board, Clothing and Lodging of Nurses, and Rest and Relaxation of Nurses. The hospitals visited by the Committee were Sir Patrick Dun's Hospital, the City of Dublin Hospital, Dr Steevens' Hospital, the Meath Hospital, Mercer's Hospital, Whitworth Hospital (Drumcondra), the Coombe Lying-in Hospital, the Rotunda Lying-in Hospital, St Mark's Ophthalmic Hospital, the National Eye and Ear Infirmary, Cork Street Fever Hospital, the Adelaide Hospital, Rathdown Hospital, and the Dublin Orthopaedic Hospital.
13 Ibid.
14 Ibid., p. 12.
15 Ibid. (original emphasis).

16　Ibid.
17　Ibid., p. 13.
18　Ibid., pp. 13–4. This specific proposal may have provided the template for both the Dublin Nurses' Training Institution, founded by Eliza Browne at 26 Usher's Quay in 1882, and the Dublin Metropolitan Technical School for Nurses, founded by Margaret Huxley in 1894.
19　Ibid.
20　Ibid.
21　DHSF, 1880, p. 34.
22　Wickham, 2000, p. 14.
23　DHSF, 1880, p. 36.
24　Ibid., p. 13.
25　Ibid.
26　Wickham, 2001, p. 33.
27　DHSF, 1881, pp. 17–21.
28　The Committee of Distribution was concerned that any immediate reduction of funds could hinder rather than advance nursing reform.
29　Gatenby, 1996, p. 171.
30　DHSF, 1883, p. 18.
31　Gatenby, 1996, p. 171.
32　For the year 1884–1885, the united income of all the Dublin hospitals was calculated to be approximately £50,000, of which £3,557 7s. 8d. was contributed by the Fund. While this contribution represented only approximately 7 per cent of the total income of all the Dublin hospitals in the year in question, it was approaching half that of the Parliamentary grant of £9,456 18s. See DHSF, 1887, p. xlvii.
33　DHSF, 1887, p. xxxvii.
34　Wickham, 2000, p. 1.
35　DHSF, 1889, p. 46.
36　DHSF, 1931.
37　The Sweepstakes was introduced by the Cumann na nGaedheal Government in 1930 in an effort to provide an urgent source of funding for a number of named hospitals in Dublin. See Daly, 1999, pp. 234–52.
38　HC, 1856 [2063], xix.115, p. 10.
39　HC, 1887a, p. i.
40　For this reason, the Commission was sometimes referred to as the 'Blennerhassett Commission'.
41　Among the voluntary hospitals that were the subject of the Commission's inquiries were the Mater Misericordiae Hospital, the Charitable Infirmary, the Dublin House of Industry Hospitals, Dr Steevens' Hospital, Sir Patrick Dun's Hospital, Mercer's Hospital and the City of Dublin Hospital.
42　Ibid., p. 124 (evidence of Mr Christopher J. Nixon).
43　Ibid., p. 129 (evidence of Dr Thomas More Madden).
44　Ibid., p. 140 (evidence of Mr Arthur Chance).
45　Ibid., p. 134 (evidence of Mr Edward Thomas Stapleton).
46　Meehan, 2003, pp. 99–107.
47　Fahey, 1987, p. 7–30.
48　Ibid.
49　Nelson, 2001.
50　HC, 1887a, p. xxxv.
51　Ibid., p. 148 (evidence of Rev. Samuel Haughton). This is an apparent reference to evidence given in respect of the Dublin House of Industry Hospitals where, it seems, elderly nurses were employed.
52　Ibid.
53　Ibid., p. 117 (evidence of Mr H. Gray Croly).

54   Ibid., p. 118 (evidence of Mr William Ireland Wheeler).
55   Ibid., p. 64 (evidence of Mr F. Alcock Nixon) and p. 170 (evidence of Dr C. F. Knight).
56   Ibid., p. 69 (evidence of Mr Edward Stamer O'Grady).
57   Ibid., p. 84 (evidence of Mr Abraham Shackleton).
58   Ibid., p. 2 (evidence of Mr William Stokes), p. 6 (evidence of Dr W. Thompson) and p. 30 (evidence of Mr John M. Prior Kennedy).
59   Ibid., p. 90 (evidence of Arthur V. Macan).
60   Ibid., p. xix.
61   Ibid., p. li.
62   The central fund would be known as the Educational Endowment, since medical education would remain the principal grounds for the continuance of the Parliamentary grant.
63   HC, 1887a, pp. lii–liii.
64   HC, 1887b (302) ii.191. In 1889, a second bill proposing the establishment of a Dublin Hospital Board was published. See HC, 1889 (389), i.585.
65   DHSF, 1888, p. 11.
66   The Bill did not receive any further mention in subsequent annual reports of the Council of the Fund.
67   Scanlan, 1991, p. 77.
68   HC, 1858 [2353], xxiii.533.
69   HC, 1890 [C.6037], xxxii.670, p. 8.
70   While the Charitable Infirmary Jervis Street was founded within the Protestant tradition of philanthropy, its nursing arrangements were under the supervision of the Sisters of Mercy. The Mater Misericordiae and St Vincent's hospitals provided clinical training for the Catholic University Medical School.
71   Daly, 1999, pp. 234–52.
72   Wickham, 2001, p. 30.
73   Ibid., p. 26.
74   Ibid.

3   Hospitals in transition

1   By 1875, eight of the twelve teaching hospitals in London had a nurse training institution. See Helmstadter, 2003, pp. 2–30.
2   House of Commons (hereafter cited as HC), 1887a [C.5042], xxxv.1, p. xxxvi.
3   Ibid., p. 223 (evidence of Lord Justice FitzGibbon).
4   Dublin Hospital Sunday Fund, hereafter cited as DHSF, 1879, p. 5.
5   City of Dublin Hospital (hereafter cited as CDH), 1879, p. 7.
6   Board of Directors Minute Book, CDH, 1879, p. 36.
7   Ibid., 4 April 1879, p. 40.
8   CDH, 1880, p. 6.
9   Board of Directors Minute Book, CDH, 8 June 1883, p. 184.
10   Ibid., 16 November 1883, p. 207.
11   CDH, 1884a, p. 8.
12   Board of Directors Minute Book, CDH, 16 November 1883, p. 211.
13   CDH, 1884b, pp. 222–5.
14   Ibid., p. 222.
15   Board of Directors Minute Book, CDH, 8 February 1884c, p. 227.
16   Ibid., 15 February 1884, p. 229.
17   CDH, 1884d, pp. 232–3.
18   Board of Directors Minute Book, CDH, 18 April 1884c.
19   Ibid., pp. 242–4.
20   Ibid., p. 243.

21   CDH, 1885, p. 7.
22   Board of Directors Minute Book, CDH, 18 April 1884c, pp. 246–7.
23   CDH, 1886, p. 10.
24   CDH, 1887, p. 10.
25   CDH, 1886, p. 10.
26   CDH, 1888, p. 9.
27   Anon., 1892, p. 5.
28   Ibid.
29   CDH, 1892, p. 10.
30   CDH, 1894, p. 10.
31   Unidentified newspaper cutting dated 29 December 1899 (Insert in Board of Directors Minute Book, CDH, December 1899).
32   CDH, 1903, p. 10.
33   CDH, 1911, p. 10.
34   Widdess, 1972, p. 3.
35   HC, 1887a, p. iii.
36   Ibid., p. ii. Because of its status as an institution wholly funded by Parliament, the Dublin House of Industry was sometimes referred to as the 'Government Hospitals'.
37   The names of the various hospitals were derived from the names of the Viceroys – the Earl of Hardwicke, the Earl of Whitworth, and the Duke of Richmond – who were in office at the time of their opening. See Widdess, 1972, p. 7.
38   Widdess, 1972, p. 7 and pp. 132–6; HC, 1887a, p. v.
39   HC, 1854 (383), p. 110 (evidence of Dr E. Hutton). The Richmond Hospital (Medical) School was established in 1826 and in 1848 it became the Carmichael School of Medicine.
40   Ibid., p. iii and p. 251 (evidence of George James Guthrie).
41   Ibid., p. 206 (evidence of Dr Dominic Corrigan).
42   Minutes of Proceedings of the Board of Governors, Dublin House of Industry Hospitals (hereafter cited as DHIH), 10 August 1871, p. 10.
43   HC, 1854, p. 207 (evidence of Dr Dominic Corrigan).
44   Clery, 1972, pp. 155–63.
45   HC, 1887a, p. 37 (evidence of Mr William Thornley Stoker).
46   Minutes of Proceedings of the Board of Governors, DHIH, 10 August 1871, p. 10.
47   Ibid., 12 May 1881, p. 100.
48   The Chairman of the Dublin Hospitals Commission visited the Hospital on 15 June 1885.
49   Minutes of Proceedings of the Board of Governors, DHIH, 24 September 1885, p. 52.
50   Ibid., 9 March 1888, p. 1.
51   Ibid., p. 2.
52   Ibid.
53   Ibid.
54   Ibid.
55   'Matron's Explanation Relative to Report Supplied to her by Mr. Hughes by Direction of Governors, 19th March 1888' (Insert in Minutes of Proceedings of the Board of Governors, DHIH, 10 May 1888, p. 269).
56   Ibid.
57   Ibid. (original emphases).
58   Minutes of Proceedings of the Board of Governors, DHIH, 10 May 1888, p. 269.
59   Minutes of Proceedings of the Board of Governors, DHIH, 9 August 1888, p. 293.
60   Ibid., 11 April 1889, p. 376.
61   Ibid.
62   Ibid., 11 June 1889, pp. 391–2.
63   HC, 1890 [C.5751], xxxii.533, p. 6.

64 HC, 1892 [C.6729], xxxiii.539, p. 8.
65 Minutes of Proceedings of the Board of Governors, DHIH, 24 November 1892, p. 237.
66 Ibid., 8 February 1894, p. 332.
67 Miss Hughes went on to take up the position of Lady Superintendent of the Richmond Lunatic Asylum at Portrane, Co. Dublin.
68 Anon., 1909, p. 6
69 Anon., 1896d, p. 6.
70 Widdess, 1972, p. 163.
71 HC, 1899 [C. 9364] xxix.175, pp. 10–1.
72 Anon., 1902, pp. 27, 28 and 30.
73 Ibid.
74 Ibid., p. 28.
75 Widdess, 1972, p. 163.
76 Anon., 1909, p. 6.
77 Anon., 1902, p. 27.
78 McGann, 1992, p. 130.
79 Anon., 1902, p. 27.
80 Arden, 2002, p. 43.
81 Ibid., pp. 43–55.
82 Ibid., pp. 43 and 56.
83 Ibid., p. 43.
84 Fealy, 2005, pp. 23–47.
85 Arden, 2002, p. 43.
86 Summers, 2000, p. 93.
87 D'Antonio, 1997, pp. 16–7.
88 Summers, 1989b, pp. 365–86.
89 Helmstadter, 2003, pp. 2–30.
90 Witz, 1992.

4 The lady nurses of the Dublin hospitals

1 Costello, 1897, p. 7.
2 See Simonton, 2001, pp. 35–47.
3 Cited in Digby and Searby, 1981, p. 207.
4 Raftery, 1997, p. 13.
5 Spender (ed.), 1987, p. 5.
6 Purvis, 1989, p. 53.
7 Simonton, 2001, p. 41.
8 Romanes, 1987, pp. 10–36.
9 Cited in Raftery, 1997, p. 152.
10 Purvis, 1989, pp. 48 and 224.
11 Raftery, 1997, p. 16.
12 Borer contends that the quality of education in the middle-class finishing schools was poor, with private governesses having no training to teach. See Borer, 1975.
13 Purvis, 1989, p. 93.
14 Ibid., pp. 197–8.
15 O'Connor, 1987, pp. 31–54.
16 Spender, 1987, p. 6; Raftery, 1997, p. 123.
17 Purvis, 1989, p. 225. Purvis is here referring to working-class women's struggle to gain access to educational institutes in England that were initially established as part of the mechanical institutes and the workingmen's college movement.
18 Digby and Searby, 1981, pp. 49 and 209.
19 Tod, 1987, pp. 230–47.
20 Jex-Blake, 1987, pp. 268–76.

21   Breathnach, 1987, pp. 55–78.
22   O'Connor, 1987, pp. 31–54.
23   O'Connor, 1995, pp. 125–59.
24   Breathnach, 1987, pp. 58–9; O' Connor, 1995, p. 139.
25   O'Connor, 1987, p. 50.
26   Scott, 1993, pp. 399–426.
27   Ibid.
28   O'Connor, 1995, pp. 143–4.
29   Ibid.
30   Anon., 1895b, p. 5.
31   Rafferty, 1996, p. 42.
32   Rafferty, 1995, pp. 43–56.
33   Bradshaw, 2001, p. 10 and p. 14.
34   Lorentzon, 2003, pp. 325–31.
35   Ibid., pp. 327–8
36   Meehan, 2003, pp. 99–107; See also Summers, 2000, p. 81; Nelson, 1997, pp. 6–14.
37   See Helmstadter, 2003, pp. 2–30.
38   Helmstadter, 1997, p. 161–197. The original name of St John's House was 'The Training Institution for Nurses, for Hospitals, Families and the Sick Poor'. For a detailed discussion of the contribution of Robert Bentley Todd to nursing reform, see Helmstadter, 1993a, pp. 282–319. The St John's House model was itself indirectly influenced by the earlier nineteenth-century movement for the reformation of manners in the English upper-class public schools, reforms that also stressed moral and religious (Christian) education, or 'character building'. See Helmstadter, 2003, p. 8.
39   Rafferty, 1995, p. 43; Helmstadter, 1993b, pp. 43–70.
40   Rafferty, 1996, p. 58.
41   Abel-Smith, 1960, p. 21.
42   Helmstadter, 1993b, pp. 43–70.
43   Rafferty, 1996, p. 52.
44   Kirkpatrick, 1924, pp. 281–2. See also Scanlan, 1991, p. 72. The precise date of the establishment of the Institution is unclear. Kirkpatrick offers conflicting dates. In his history of Dr Steevens' Hospital, he suggests that the date was sometime after 1864 and before 1866. In another publication, Kirkpatrick places the year of the founding of the Institution as 1860. See Kirkpatrick, 1917a, pp. 14–5.
45   Scanlan, 1991, pp. 72–3.
46   Kirkpatrick, 1917a, pp. 14–5.
47   Anon., 1895b, p. 5.
48   Coakley, 1995, p. 29. The City of Dublin Hospital, Baggot Street became the Royal City of Dublin Hospital in 1900 when it was granted a Royal Charter.
49   Anon., 1896a, p. 5.
50   Scanlan, 1991, p. 75. See also Anon., 1895d, p. 5.
51   McGann, 1992, p. 135. For a detailed study of the Dublin Metropolitan Technical School for Nurses, see Fealy, 2005, pp. 23–47. See also *Irish Nursing News* 1928, Vol. VII (11), p. 139.
52   Scanlan, 1991, p. 81.
53   Costello, 1897, pp. 7–8.
54   Bradshaw, 2001, p. 14. For a discussion on the functions and features of the dual probationership system, see Brooks, 2001, pp. 13–21. See also Weir, 2000, pp. 42–7.
55   Richmond, Whitworth and Hardwicke Hospitals, 1890.
56   Anon., 1985d, p. 5.
57   Proceedings of Minutes of the Governing Authority, Dublin Metropolitan Technical School for Nurses, 5 January 1894.
58   Anon., 1895a, p. 7.
59   Anon., 1896c, p. 6.

60 Anon., 1895c, p. 5.
61 McNeill, 1934, p. 127.
62 Anon., 1894, p. 5. *The Lady of the House* uses the term 'Institute' in the title of its article. The minutes of the proceedings from the Board of Governors of the City of Dublin Hospital, indicate the use of the term 'Institution'; Anon., 1895d, p. 5.
63 Anon.,1895e, pp. 5–6; Anon., 1895h, p. 4; Anon., 1895a, p. 7.
64 Anon., 1895h, p. 4.
65 Nolan, 1991, p. 10.
66 Anon., 1896d, p. 6.
67 Anon., 1896a, p. 5.
68 Anon., 1896b, p. 7.
69 Ibid.
70 Nolan, 1991, p. 12.
71 Ibid., pp. 8–13.
72 Anon., 1894, p. 5.
73 Anon., 1985e, p. 5.
74 Anon., 1895g, p. 7.
75 Anon., 1895d p. 5.
76 Anon., 1895a, p. 7.
77 Anon., 1895d, p. 5.
78 Anon., 1895g, p. 7 (original emphasis).
79 Anon., 1895f, pp. 3–4.
80 Anon., 1896b, p. 7; Anon., 1895g, p. 7.
81 Anon., 1894, p. 5; Anon., 1986b, p. 7.
82 Barber, 1998, pp. 20–9. See also Pearson *et al.*, 2001, pp. 147–52.
83 Anon., 1895a, p. 7.
84 Anon., 1896c, p. 6.
85 Anon., 1895g, p. 7.
86 Anon., 1896a, p. 5.
87 Barber, 1998, pp. 21–2.
88 Ibid., p. 26.
89 Pearson *et al.*, 2001, p. 147.
90 Anon., 1985d, p. 5; Anon., 1895a, p. 7.
91 Barber, 1998, p. 27.
92 Rumsey, 1873, p. 4 (available at Library of Trinity College Dublin).
93 Anon., 1895b, p. 5.
94 Brooks, 2001, pp. 13–21.
95 Coakley, 1995, p. 31.
96 Nolan, 1991, p. 13.
97 McGann, 1992, p. 137.
98 Costello, 1897, pp. 7–8.
99 Ibid., p. 8.
100 Connolly and Ryan, 2000.
101 Helmstadter, 1993b, pp. 43–70.
102 Lorentzon, 2001, pp. 4–12.
103 Ibid., p. 10.

5 Professional regulation and the General Nursing Council for Ireland

1 House of Commons, hereafter cited as HC, 1919a; HC, 1919b, 9 &10, c. 96.
2 Hector, 1973, p. 34.
3 The 'thirty years' refers to the period between 1888, when the British Nurses' Association was founded, and 1919, when the Nurses' Registration Act was passed. See Abel-Smith, 1960, p. 67. For an examination of the ideologies that underpinned

the opposing positions in the registration debate, see Rafferty, 1996, pp. 42–67. See also Rafferty, 1993, pp. 48–60. For an examination of the role of Mrs Bedford Fenwick in the registration movement, see Hector, 1973. For a summary and discussion of the arguments for and against state registration that were put to the Select Committee on the Registration of Nurses, 1904–1905, see Bradshaw, 2001, pp. 76–7.

4   McGann, 1992, p. 141.
5   HC, 1904a (281) vi.701 and 1905 (263) vii.301, p. 22 (evidence of Margaret Huxley).
6   Bradshaw, 2001, p. 66.
7   Griffon, 1995, pp. 201–12.
8   Ibid., p. 203.
9   Rafferty, 1996, p. 65.
10 Abel-Smith, 1960, p. 93.
11 Rafferty, 1996, p. 66.
12 Dingwall, Rafferty, and Webster, 1988, p. 81.
13 Witz, 1992, p. 137. Witz points out that private duty nurses comprised nearly three-quarters of the nursing workforce up to 1914.
14 Ibid.
15 Griffon, 1995, p. 204.
16 McGann, 1992, pp. 38–9.
17 Baly, 1995, p. 146.
18 Bradshaw, 2001, p. 57.
19 Griffon, 1995, p. 206.
20 Abel-Smith, 1960, p. 66.
21 Rafferty, 1993, p. 55.
22 Bradshaw, 2001, p. 58.
23 Scanlan, 1991, p. 87.
24 McGann, 1992, pp. 137–8.
25 Ibid.
26 HC, 1904a, p. iii.
27 Ibid., p. 21 (evidence of Margaret Huxley).
28 For a detailed discussion of the role of Huxley as a lobbyist, see McGann, 1992, pp. 141–3. Huxley acted as President of the National Council of Trained Nurses of Great Britain and Ireland for the year 1913.
29 The Central Committee for the State Registration of Nurses was an association of pro-registration societies, formed following Mr Asquith's refusal in 1909 to allow the Nurses' Registration Bill to be debated in the House of Commons. See Abel-Smith, 1960, p. 82.
30 Reeves, 1940, pp. 27–8.
31 Abel-Smith, 1960, pp. 87–9.
32 McGann, 1992, p. 146; Scanlan, 1991, p. 89.
33 The members of the Irish Board of the College of Nursing included Miss Eddison (Royal City of Dublin Hospital), Miss Hill (Adelaide Hospital), Miss McGivney (Mater Misericordiae Hospital), and Miss Phelan (South Dublin Union). Its members from outside of Dublin included Miss Bostock (Royal Victoria Hospital, Belfast), Miss Curtin (the Mater Hospital, Belfast), Miss Coffey (Barrington's Hospital, Limerick) and Miss McDowell (Waterford County Infirmary). See McGann, 1992, pp. 146–7.
34 McGann, 1992, pp. 144–9.
35 *British Medical Journal*, 24 March 1917.
36 McGann, 1992, p. 147. The members of the Irish Nursing Board included Miss Bradburne (Meath Hospital), Miss Hezlett (Richmond Hospital), Miss Jordan (Mercer's Hospital), Miss Reeves (Dr Steevens' Hospital), Miss Sutton (St Vincent's Hospital), Miss Thornton (Sir Patrick Dun's Hospital), Miss Carson Rae (Cork Street Fever Hospital), Miss Ramsden (Rotunda Hospital), Miss Keating (National

Maternity Hospital), Miss O'Flynn (the Children's Hospital Temple Street) and Miss West (North Dublin Union).

37 Kirkpatrick, 1917b, p. 7. See also Scanlan, 1991, p. 89.
38 *British Medical Journal*, 24 March 1917. Nurses who had entered training on or before July 1917 could have their names enrolled on the register for a fee of one guinea.
39 Kirkpatrick, 1917b, p. 7.
40 Ibid.
41 Ibid., p. 3.
42 HC, 1904b, 59 (iii), 593.
43 Abel-Smith, 1960, pp. 81–2.
44 Ibid., p. 96.
45 HC, 1919b, 9 & 10, c. 94.
46 McGann, 1992, p. 151.
47 The bill provided for a membership of ten initially, to include four persons appointed by the Chief Secretary and six persons who were nurse members, but this was increased to fifteen upon an amendment to the bill.
48 HC, 1919b, Clause 3, para. 1.
49 Minutes of General Nursing Council for Ireland (hereafter cited as GNCI), February 1920 – December 1943, Minutes 25 February 1920.
50 Ibid., 17 June 1920.
51 Miss Huxley, Miss O'Flynn, Miss Reeves and Miss Michie represented the Irish Nursing Board, while the members of the Irish Board of the College of Nursing were Mrs Bostock, Miss Curtin and Miss Metheson. The latter body was dissolved in 1925, although its parent body, the College of Nursing, went on to attain a royal charter in 1939 and it expanded as an independent professional body for nursing, midwifery and health visiting in the United Kingdom. Sir Arthur Chance was the Chairman of the Irish Nursing Board. See McGann, 1992, pp. 152–3. The two other nursing members of the Council were Miss Margaret Walsh, Matron of Mosaphir Private Nursing Home, Cork, and Mrs Mary Blunden, Matron of the Waterford Union Infirmary. The three representatives of the Council from the six counties of Ulster ceased to become members when the Joint Nursing Council for Nursing and Midwifery for Northern Ireland was established.
52 Minutes GNCI, 1 June 1920. The Rules Committee comprised Colonel Taylor, Miss Huxley, Miss Reeves, Miss Matheson and Miss O'Flynn.
53 Ibid. The Rules established the sixth standard of education or its equivalent as 'a sufficient standard' of education.
54 GNCI, Rules Made Under Nurses' Registration (Ireland) Act 1919, Dublin: General Nursing Council for Ireland, 1920, Article II, parts 1 and 2.
55 Ibid., Article IV, part 2.
56 HC, 1919b. Section 3 (2c) of the Act made provision for such an eventuality.
57 Minutes GNCI, 25 February 1920 (Report of the Finance Committee).
58 Ibid., February 25, 1921 (Report of the Rules Committee). The Rules Committee redrafted the Rules, omitting the clause that precluded the admittance of persons who had not received a minimum of one year's training.
59 Minutes GNCI, 17 June 1920.
60 Ibid., 9 March 1922.
61 Ibid., 21 October 1920.
62 GNCI, 1923; Minutes, GNCI, 19 July 1923.
63 The regulations pertaining to hospitals training nurses for admission only to the Supplementary Part of the Register related to male nurses, mental nurses, sick children's nurses, and fever nurses.
64 Minutes GNCI, 14 November 1923 (Report of the Rules Committee).
65 McGann, 1992, p. 153. The General Nursing Council for Ireland initially opposed the establishment of a General Nursing Council for Northern Ireland, on the grounds

that it would 'seriously interfere with the interests of nurse … [and] occasion much extra trouble for Nurses who may be desirous of acting throughout the entire country'. See Minutes GNCI, 9 March 1922.

66   For a discussion of the process by which the first Dáil Éireann assumed control of local government in the area of medical relief, see Barrington, 1987, Chapter 5.

67   Barrington, 1987, p. 95. In 1924, under the Ministers and Secretaries Act, the new department became the Department of Local Government and Public Health. The fact that the new Irish Free State had responsibility for the regulation of nursing in Ireland became explicit in the appearance of 'Saorstat Éireann' (Irish Free State) on the General Nursing Council's official documents in 1924. The General Nursing Council for Ireland was responsible to the Minister for Local Government.

68   Daly, 1999, pp. 234–52.

69   Barrington, 1987, p. 96.

70   McGann, 1992, p. 154. See also Minutes GNCI, 22 February 1924. Coincidentally, Mrs Bedford Fenwick also lost her seat in the first election of the General Nursing Council for England and Wales in 1923.

71   Sir Edward Coey Bigger continued to be unanimously re-elected to the post of Chairman of the Council and remained in the post until his death in 1934. See Robins, 2000a, pp. 11–27.

72   Minutes GNCI, 22 February 1924.

73   Ibid., 19 February 1929. Under the Council of 1929, new committees were appointed, including committees for Hospitals, Rules, Registration, Finance, and Uniform and Badge committees. A new Penal Cases Committee comprising the entire membership of the Council was also established and an Advisory Committee on Mental Nursing was appointed to monitor the appointments of persons as mental nurses. Sir Edward was now a member of the Irish Senate.

74   Senator Sir Edward Coey Bigger was again elected as Council Chairman, although on this occasion, a second candidate Dr Patrick MacCarville was nominated and received the votes of four of the ten members present at the new Council's first meeting in February 1934. See Minutes GNCI, 1 February 1934.

75   Minutes GNCI, 23 March 1926.

76   For a discussion of the relationship of the voluntary hospitals with the new Free State Government during the inter-war years, see Daly, 1999, pp. 234–52.

77   Minutes GNCI, 25 August 1925.

78   Ibid., 18 October 1927.

79   Ibid., 19 March 1931. Alice Reeves was elected to the Council in April 1930, when a vacancy arose. It is unclear if this vacancy arose from the ill health of the Council member Miss O'Flynn, or from the apparent inability of another member, Miss Buckley, to procure leave from her employers to attend meetings of the Council. See Minutes GNCI, 26 November 1931.

80   The number of candidates in Dublin far exceeded the total number of candidates in the rest of the country.

81   GNCI, 1934.

82   GNCI, 1931.

83   Among the hospitals to apply for approval were Barrington's Hospital, Limerick; Clonmel District Mental Hospital; and Belmont Park Institution, Waterford.

84   Minutes GNCI, 18 November 1936.

85   The 'affiliated training schools' were Meath County Infirmary, Navan, affiliated to Sir Patrick Dun's Hospital; the County Hospital Wexford and St John's Hospital, Limerick, both affiliated to the Mercy Hospital, Cork; Our Lady of Lourdes, Dublin, affiliated to Dr Steevens' and Mercer's hospitals; and St Mary's Hospital, Cappagh, affiliated to St Vincent's Hospital and the Royal City of Dublin Hospital. The three 'amalgamated training schools' were the County Hospital Waterford with the County and City Infirmary Waterford; Barrington's Hospital, Limerick with the County

Infirmary, Limerick; and Drumcondra Hospital, Dublin with Mayo County Hospital, Castlebar.
86 Minutes GNCI, 11 March 1936.
87 Ibid., 16 June 1937.
88 Ibid., 9 December 1937.
89 Kirkpatrick, 1917b, p. 4.
90 For a discussion on nursing's involvement in the women's movement during the first decade of the twentieth century, see S. Lewenson, 1994, pp. 99–117.
91 Griffon, 1995, p. 205.
92 Abel-Smith, 1960, p. 67.
93 Hector, 1973, p. 39.
94 Bradshaw, 2001, pp. 76–7.
95 Robins, 2000a, p. 20.

6 'Knowledge of her work'

1 Cantlie, 1914, p. 1.
2 Pincoffs, 1893, pp. 45–6.
3 Minutes of Proceedings of the Governing Authority, Dublin Metropolitan Technical School for Nurses (hereafter cited as DMTSN), 16 December 1893–19 May 1952 (Minutes, 5 January 1894).
4 Rafferty, 1996, p. 11.
5 Anderson, 1897, pp. 5–6.
6 Ibid., pp. 5–6 and 10–11.
7 Anon., 1895c, p. 5.
8 Scanlan, 1991, p. 106.
9 Ibid., pp. 107–8.
10 Ibid.
11 Nightingale, 1969; Lückes, 1886; Lückes, 1892; Drew, 1889.
12 Anderson, 1897; Cantlie, 1914.
13 For a list of the earliest textbooks, see *The American Journal of Nursing*, 1900, vol. 1 (1), p. 6.
14 Rafferty, 1996, p. 29.
15 Ibid., p. 33.
16 Ibid., p. 45.
17 Kirkpatrick, 1917a, pp. 15–19.
18 Ibid., pp. 18–27.
19 Anne Marie Rafferty questions the extent to which textbooks were successful in delineating the division of labour among occupationally different groups and observes that, in the clinical setting, role boundaries among doctors and nurses were not immutable. Rafferty, 1996, p. 29.
20 Gamarnikow, 1991, p. 110–129; Rafferty, 1996, p. 11.
21 Kirkpatrick, 1917a, p. 36. Here the writer is referring to the nursing of private cases, where the nurse might be more likely to have to make autonomous clinical decisions.
22 Drew, 1889, p. 24.
23 Ibid., p. 72.
24 Rafferty, 1996, p. 29.
25 Kirkpatrick, 1917a, p. 32.
26 Drew, 1889, p. 72.
27 Cantlie, 1914, p. 63.
28 Minutes of Proceedings of the Governing Authority, DMTSN, 16 December 1893.
29 The members of the first Governing Authority were Miss Huxley and Dr C. B. Ball MD (representing Sir Patrick Dun's Hospital), Miss Kelly and Dr R. A. Hayes MD (representing Dr Steevens' Hospital), Miss McDonnell and Sir William Thompson

(representing the Richmond, Whitworth and Hardwicke Hospitals), and Miss Shelley and Mr R. L. Swan (representing the Dublin Orthopaedic Hospital).

30   Minutes of Proceedings of the Governing Authority, DMTSN, 24 November 1894.
31   Ibid., 14 November 1894.
32   Fealy, 2005, vol. 13, pp. 23–47.
33   Ibid., p.39
34   Among the hospitals participating in the School's programme were the original participating hospitals, as well as the Meath, Adelaide and Mercers hospitals, the Children's Hospital Temple Street, Cork Street Fever Hospital and, latterly, the Royal City of Dublin Hospital.
35   The premises at 101 St Stephen's Green were also the premises of St Patrick's Home for supplying trained nurses to the sick poor in their own homes.
36   Minutes of the General Nursing Council for Ireland (hereafter cited as GNCI), February 1920–December 1943, (Minutes 11 March 1936).
37   Coey Bigger, 1937, pp. 45–7.
38   Richmond, Whitworth and Hardwicke Hospitals, undated, *c.* 1930.
39   Ibid.
40   Ibid., p. 8.
41   Sears, 1941.
42   *Irish Nursing News,* 1931, vol. ix (7), p. 109. In June 1931, *Irish Nursing News* published 'model answers' to the State examination questions. See *Irish Nursing News,* 1931, vol. ix (9), p. 138. The example cited was for the General Part of the Register. The general format of the examination paper for the Preliminary Examination remained constant throughout the period up to 1949.
43   *The Irish Nurses' Magazine,* 1940, vol. 10 (10), p. 7.
44   *Irish Nursing News,* 1931, vol. ix (7), p. 109; *The Irish Nurses' Magazine,* 1939, vol. 10 (3), p. 8.
45   *The Irish Nurses' Magazine,* 1939, vol. 10 (3), p. 8.
46   *The Irish Nurses' Magazine,* 1942, vol. 12 (20), p. 6.
47   Millard, 1944, pp. 6–8.
48   At the Glasgow Royal Infirmary, a preliminary training school system was established in 1893. See Weir, 2000, pp. 42–47. As early as 1920 at the Royal City of Dublin Hospital, probationers undertook a period of planned theoretical instruction before they entered the wards of the hospital and this system was referred to as the 'preliminary training school'. See Royal City of Dublin Hospital (hereafter cited as RCDH), 1920.
49   At Dublin's Mater Misericordiae Hospital, the system of morning and evening lectures appears to have been in place until the mid-1960s. See Nolan, 1991, p. 77.
50   *Irish Nursing News,* 1944, vol. XXIII, (11–12), p. 3. A preliminary training school, functioning 'along altogether different lines', operated at Sir Patrick Dun's Hospital before 1944, but it had been long since discontinued. See Sir Patrick Dun's Hospital, 1945, pp. 7–8.
51   Sir Patrick Dun's Hospital, hereafter cited as SPDH, 1945, pp. 7–8.
52   SPDH, 1946, p. 7.
53   Ibid.
54   SPDH, 1946, p. 7.
55   During the period, economic hardship was related to a number of factors, including the Economic War with Britain in the 1930s and the Second World War in the 1940s.
56   RCDH, *Nursing Committee Minute Book,* 1920.
57   *Irish Nursing News,* 1944, vol. XXIII (11–12), p. 3.
58   *The Irish Nurses' Magazine,* 1944, vol. 13 (33), p. 2.
59   Ibid.
60   The ratio of 2:1 is derived from figures presented by Pauline Scanlan. In the general training hospitals, the figures were 751 trainees to 474 qualified nurses. In 1945, out of

a total nursing workforce of 5,228, the number of nurses in training was 1,136. See Scanlan, 1991, p. 127. See also *The Irish Nurses' Magazine*, 1946, vol. 13 (61), p. 4.
61 *The Irish Nurses' Magazine*, 1943, vol. 12 (21), pp. 6–7.
62 Scanlan, 1991, p. 129.
63 Counihan, 1951, pp. 304–15. St Laurence's Hospital was the former Richmond, Whitworth and Hardwicke Hospitals.
64 *The Irish Nurses' Magazine*, 1944, vol. 13 (36), pp. 5–12.
65 Ibid., p. 5; Millard, 1944, p. 7.
66 Ibid., p. 8.
67 *Irish Nursing News*, 1944, vol. 13 (36), pp. 5–12.
68 Millard, 1944, p. 7.
69 *Irish Nursing News*, December 1948–January 1949, vol. xxvi (3–4), p. 1.
70 Cited in Robins, 2000b, p. 30.
71 *The Irish Nurses' Magazine*, 1948, vol. 15 (8), p. 2.
72 Scanlan, 1991, p. 111.

7 The Nursing Board and the training experience, 1950–1979
1 McShane, 1999, p. 41.
2 The state hospital building programme of the 1930s provided more than forty hospitals up to the outbreak of the Second World War. After the war, the programme of hospital building resumed, now funded largely by the Irish Hospitals Sweepstakes. By 1965, more than two hundred small and large hospitals had been constructed. See Deeny, 1989, p. 140.
3 Barrington, 1987, Chapter 8.
4 Robins, 2000a, p. 24. Within the new Department of Health, nursing was regarded as a 'medical ancillary service'. See *The Irish Nurses Magazine*, 1949, vol. 16 (11), pp. 2–5.
5 Barrington, 1987, p. 195. Under the Inter-party Government, Margaret F. Reidy was appointed as the first Nursing Officer in the Department of Health. See *The Irish Nurses' Magazine*, 1949, vol. 16 (8), p. 13.
6 Ibid., pp. 201–13.
7 Ibid., Chapters 8 and 9.
8 *The Irish Nurses' Magazine*, 1953, vol. 20 (2), p. 16; *The Irish Nurses' Magazine*, 1953, vol. 20 (4), p. 9. For a detailed analysis of this episode in Irish politics, see Barrington, 1987, Chapter 8. See also Whyte, 1971.
9 Barrington, 1987, pp. 247–50.
10 Ibid.
11 *The Irish Nurses' Magazine*, 1948, vol. 15 (4), p. 1.
12 *The Irish Nurses' Magazine*, 1948, vol. 15 (8), pp. 1–2.
13 Ibid.
14 Government of Ireland, 1949.
15 *The Irish Nurses' Magazine*, 1949, vol. 16 (8), p. 1.
16 *The Irish Nurses' Magazine*, 1949, vol. 16 (9), pp. 1–2.
17 *The Irish Nurses' Magazine*, 1950, vol. 17 (11), p. 4.
18 Deeny, 1949, pp. 2–5.
19 Ibid.
20 The separate disciplinary procedures were provided for in the establishment of a Maternity Nurses' Committee to deal with disciplinary problems 'peculiar to maternity nursing'. See *The Irish Nurses' Magazine*, 1949, vol. 16 (8), pp. 1–2.
21 *The Irish Nurses' Magazine*, 1949, vol. 16 (9), pp. 2–3.
22 Robins, 2000b, pp. 29–30.
23 Acts of the Oireachtas, 1950, p. 13.
24 Minutes of General Nursing Council for Ireland, Minutes of An Bord Altranais General Meetings, Committees of Board, Sub-Committee Rules, Midwives

Examination Committee etc., 20 October 1945–19 December, 1951 (Minutes 7 June 1951).

25   Ibid. An Taoiseach was acting as Minister for Health, following the resignation of Dr Noël Browne. See Robins, 2000b, p. 30.

26   Ibid. Dr MacCarville resigned as President in 1953 and was replaced by Dr Ninian Falkiner. Dr Falkiner was, in turn, replaced by Dr O'Connell, who held the position of President until 1960.

27   Robins, 2000b, p. 31.

28   An Bord Altranais, 1953.

29   This provision led to the establishment of a number of post-registration courses of training at a number of Dublin hospitals.

30   An Bord Altranais, 1955.

31   An Bord Altranais, undated a.

32   Ibid., pp. 7–8.

33   Ibid.

34   Ryan, 2000, p. 79.

35   *The Irish Nurses' Magazine*, 1950, vol. 17 (11), p. 1.

36   Scanlan, 1991, p. 122. The numbers cited are approximations.

37   Ryan, 2000, p. 77–99.

38   Ibid. By the mid 1970s, this number was reduced to twenty-three.

39   The combined four-year general and sick children's nurse training programme involved Our Lady's Hospital for Sick Children, St James's Hospital, James Connolly Memorial Hospital, St Laurence's Hospital and the Mater Misericordiae Hospital. St Michael's Hospital Dun Laoghaire, in association with St John of God Hospital, Stillorgan, provided a combined four-year general and psychiatric nurse training programme.

40   Robins, 2000b, p. 43. The Nurses Act 1961 provided for the election of a President of the Board for the full five-year term of office of the Board. Prior to this, the Board elected its president on an annual basis. The first President to be appointed by the Minister was Dr W. F. O'Dwyer.

41   *The Irish Nurses' Magazine*, 1950, vol. 17 (4), p. 11; *The Irish Nurses' Magazine*, 1952, vol. 19 (5), p. 5.

42   *The Irish Nurses' Magazine*, 1952, vol. 19 (3), p. 13; *The Irish Nurses' Magazine*, 1952, vol. 19 (5), p. 5; *The Irish Nurses' Magazine*, 1952, vol. 19 (7), p. 4.

43   *The Irish Nurses' Magazine*, 1954, vol. 21 (8), p. 17. See also Mater Misericordiae Hospital, 1961, pp. 21–2.

44   *The Irish Nurses' Magazine*, 1950, vol. 17 (11), p. 4 (original emphasis).

45   Lennon, 'Nursing: Ireland v. United States', *The Irish Nurses' Magazine*, 1960, vol. 27 (11), pp. 3–7.

46   Ryan, 2000, p. 79.

47   Anon., 1966, pp. 9–10.

48   *Irish Nursing News*, 1970, January–February, p. 17.

49   Scanlan, 1991, p. 178.

50   Rose, 1957, pp. 25 and 27–8.

51   Simpson, 'Satisfaction and dissatisfaction of student life', *International Nursing Review*, 1968, vol. 15 (4), pp. 329–38.

52   Mitchell, 1989, p. 102.

53   Ibid., p. 106.

54   *Irish Nursing and Hospital World*, 1966, vol. 37 (6), pp. 9–10. See also Department of Health, 1980. The term 'block' appears to have been a corruption of the term 'en bloc'.

55   Ibid.

56   Nolan, 1991, p. 77.

57   Hanrahan, 1970, p. 114.

58   Ibid., p. 115.

59 Leydon, 1972, pp. 101–2.
60 Scanlan, 1969, pp. 153–60. These findings relate to the years 1961–62.
61 Scanlan, 1991, p. 191.
62 *The Irish Nurses' Magazine*, 1962, vol. 29 (5), p. 3.
63 Ibid.
64 *The Irish Nurses' Magazine*, 1959, vol. 26 (8), p. 3.
65 Scanlan, 1991, p. 260. See also Tierney, 1974, pp. 111–7.
66 *Irish Nurses' Journal*, 1969, vol. 2 (6), p. 15.
67 Rose, 1957, p. 28.
68 Hanrahan, 1970, Chapter 5.
69 Culhane, 1952, pp. 7–8.
70 Hanrahan, 1970, p. 114.
71 Bradshaw, 2001, p. 142.
72 Mitchell, 1989, pp. 86–107.
73 Boland, 1957, pp. 24–5.
74 McGowan, 1980, p. 99.
75 Cited in Mitchell, 1989, p. 106.
76 McGowan, 1980, p. 126.
77 Chavasse, 1968, pp. 182–8.
78 An Bord Altranais, undated b.
79 Lennon, 1960, p. 4.
80 McGowan, 1980.
81 Hanrahan, 1970, p. 117.
82 Mater Misericordiae Hospital, 1961, pp. 21–2.
83 S. M. C., 1961, pp. 62–70.
84 Chavasse, 2000.
85 Boland, 1957, pp. 24–5. The building in question was the old nurses' home at St Stephen's Green; Mater Misericordiae Hospital, 1961, pp. 21–2.
86 Cited in Mitchell, 1989, p. 102.
87 Ibid.
88 Simpson, 1968, pp. 329–38.
89 Hanrahan, 1970, Chapter 5.
90 *Irish Nursing and Hospital World*, 1966, vol. 37 (6), pp. 9–10.
91 Cited in Mitchell, 1989, p. 107.
92 Hanrahan, 1970, pp. 106–7.
93 Simpson, 1968, p. 333.
94 MacGuire, 1968, vol. 19, pp. 271–82.
95 Ibid., p. 280.
96 Chavasse, 1968, pp. 182–8.
97 Ryan, 2000, p. 79.
98 Chavasse, 1968, p. 186.
99 Hanrahan, 1970, p. 81.
100 Ibid., p. 86.
101 Tierney, 1974, p. 113.
102 Royal City of Dublin Hospital, Report 1969–1975, p. 25.
103 Tierney, '1974, p. 113. An Bord Altranais introduced the minimum entry standard for nursing as a pass Leaving Certificate in 1973. See An Bord Altranais 1973.
104 Elms *et al.*, 1974, vol. 11, pp. 163–72.
105 Ibid., p. 166.
106 Dwyer and Taaffe, 1997, pp. 237–52.
107 *The Irish Nurses' Magazine*, 1955, vol. 23 (2), p. 8.
108 Maillart, 1973, vol. 154, pp. 13–6.
109 *Irish Nurses' Journal*, 1968, vol. 2 (8), p. 7.
110 Broe, 1955.

111 Ibid.
112 Scanlan, 1966, pp. 356–7.
113 Elms *et al.*, 1974, p. 166.
114 *Irish Nurses' Journal*, 1968, vol. 1 (4), p. 1.
115 Elms *et al.*, 1974, pp. 163–72.
116 *Irish Nurses' Journal*, 1969, vol. 2 (2), p. 9.
117   Rose, 1957, p. 27.

8 From the hospital to the academy, 1980–1994

1   Department of Health, 1986.
2   World Health Organization, 1985.
3   McShane, 1999, p. 82.
4   Department of Health, 1980, p. 2; Robins, 2000c, p. 57.
5   Ibid., para. 5.3, p. 83. The recommendations on minimum entry requirements proposed a minimum of two honours in the Leaving Certificate.
6   Acts of the Oireachtas, 1985; See also Robins, 2000c, p. 58.
7   Ibid., 1985, Section 36.2.
8   Quinn, 1980, pp. 168–76. See also Russell, 1980, pp. 24–5.
9   Ibid.
10   Council of the European Communities, 'Council Directive of 27 June 1977 concerning the mutual recognition of diplomas, certificates and other evidence of formal qualifications of nurses responsible for general care, including measures to facilitate the effective exercise of this right of establishment and freedom to provide services (77/452/EEC)'; 'Council Directive of 27 June 1977 concerning the co-ordination of provisions laid down by law, regulation or administrative action in respect of the activities of nurses responsible for general care (77/453.EEC)', *Official Journal of the European Communities*, 1977, vol. 20, no. L 176, pp. 1–13. The European Directives of 1977 applied only to 'nurses responsible for general care'.
11   Leydon, 1979, vol. 8 (1 and 2), p. 2.
12   Directive 77/452/EEC was concerned with criteria and mechanisms for establishing eligibility for the recognition of professional qualifications and with the duties of the host state.
13   Directive 77/453/EEC, art. 1, paras 2 b and 3.
14   Ibid., Annex.
15   An Bord Altranais, 1979.
16   An Bord Altranais, 1980.
17   The 'Proficiency Assessment Form' (PAF) permitted a rating of the student's performance in eight categories of proficiency on a five-point rating scale of performance from 'excellent' (a score of 1) to 'unsatisfactory' (a score of 5).
18   Chavasse, 2000, pp. 197–212.
19   Council of the European Communities, 'Council Directive of 10 October 1989, (89/595/EEC) amending Directives concerning the mutual recognition of diplomas, certificates and other evidence of formal qualifications of nurses responsible for general care, including measures to facilitate the effective exercise of this right of establishment and freedom to provide services, and amending Directive 77/453/EEC concerning the co-ordination of provisions laid down by law, regulation or administrative action in respect of the activities of nurses responsible for general care', *Official Journal of the European Communities*, 1989, no. L 341/30, article 2, para. 4.
20   An Bord Altranais, 1991a.
21   Simons *et al.*, 1998, p. xvii.
22   An Bord Altranais, 1994a, para. 2.7, p. 10. In 1979, the student nurse population was approximately half that of the registered nurse population in the general hospital sector. See Department of Health, 1980, p. 23.

23   Following the adoption of the first directives in 1979, it was estimated that at least one-third of the student nurses' training time was given over to meeting the requirements of the Directive. See McNamara, 1987, vol. 6 (1), pp. 3–5.

24   Department of Health, 1980, pp. 82–9.

25   An Bord Altranais, 1991b, pp. 19–21.

26   McCarthy, 1989, pp. 213–4.

27   Ibid., p. 252. McCarthy employed Cattell's Sixteen Personality Factor Test.

28   Ibid., p. 10.

29   An Bord Altranais, 1994a, para. 2.6, p. 8. On the basis of data supplied to the Working Party on General Nursing, it was calculated that each individual made an average of three applications. See An Bord Altranais, 1991b, p. 22.

30   An Bord Altranais, 1991b, p. 23.

31   An Bord Altranais, 1987, pp. 1–2.

32   Robins, 2000c, p. 60. The CAO is the national applications agency for entry to third level education in Ireland.

33   Ibid. A legal challenge to the CAB was part of the strategy of the opposition.

34   McCarthy, 1989, p. 3.

35   Robins, 2000c, p. 60.

36   An Bord Altranais, 1991b, pp. 49–50.

37   Teaching grew in popularity during the 1980s and the number of Registered Nurse Tutors increased, following the introduction of the Bachelor of Nursing Studies degree course for nurse tutor training at University College Dublin in 1984.

38   An Bord Altranais, 1994a, para. 2.8, p. 12.

39   Department of Health, 1980, para. 4.18.1, p. 61. This situation was mirrored in Britain, where there was evidence that many nurse tutors had lost touch with the reality of clinical practice. See Bendall, 1975.

40   An Bord Altranais, 1994a, para. 2.8, p. 12.

41   Department of Health, 1980, para. 4.18.2, p. 62.

42   Fealy, 1997, vol. 25, pp. 1061–69.

43   Simons *et al.*, 1998, p. xvii.

44   Cowman, 1989, vol. 7 (3 and 4), pp. 25–7.

45   Ibid., p. 27.

46   For an example of research examining the social processes involved in shaping the student nurse's experience in the UK, see Melia, 1987. For an example of research into the social processes at work in the professional socialization of the student nurse in Ireland, see Treacy, 1989, vol. 25, pp. 70–91. Treacy's research, undertaken in the mid 1980s, involved in-depth interviews with Irish student nurses, nurse tutors, ward sisters and registered nurses. All but one of the student sample of thirty-six students was female. See also Treacy, 1987, pp. 164–75.

47   Treacy, 1989, pp. 70–91.

48   Ibid., p. 88.

49   Treacy, 1987, p. 166.

50   For a discussion on the role of hierarchical structures in hospitals, see Davies, 1995. For a psychoanalytical perspective (specifically Klienian) on the organization of hospital work and hospital social systems, see Menzies Lyth, 2000, pp. 439–62.

51   Bennett, 1986, p. 20.

52   Treacy, 1987, p. 166.

53   Treacy, 1989, p. 78.

54   Simons, *et al.*, 1998, p. 37.

55   An Bord Altranais, 1991b, p. 13.

56   Simons, *et al.*, 1998, pp. 36–8.

57   *World of Irish Nursing*, 1973, vol. 2 (6), p. 101.

58   The Faculty of Nursing offered 'diploma' courses in a variety of subjects, including applied physiology, pharmacology and pathology and the Faculty also conferred a

Fellowship in Nursing. At the time, there existed a lack of clarity as to the precise status of the academic awards offered by the Faculty. See Chavasse, 2000, p. 208. See also Tierney, 1974, pp. 111–17.

59   An Bord Altranais, 1994a, para. 2.13, p. 16. The submissions were prepared by University College Galway (1979), the Midland Health Board (1984), the North-Western Health Board (1987), Waterford Regional Technical College (1987), University College Dublin (1991), and Trinity College Dublin in association with St James's Hospital and the MANCH group of hospitals (Meath, Adelaide and the National Children's hospitals) (*c*.1992).

60   McCarthy, 1990a, pp. 5–14. McCarthy later become Professor of Nursing at University College Cork.

61   Ibid., p. 12.

62   Ibid. See also McCarthy, 1990b, p. 38.

63   Cowman, 1990. Cowman later became Professor of Nursing at the Faculty of Nursing and Midwifery, Royal College of Surgeons in Ireland.

64   McNamara, 1987, p. 3.

65   Ibid., p. 4.

66   An Bord Altranais, 1991b, p. 1. The review was established in accordance with the provision of the Nurses' Act of 1985, Part IV, Section 36 (2), which conferred on the Board the responsibility to review and evaluate existing programmes of nurse training.

67   Ibid.

68   An Bord Altranais, 1994a, p. x.

69   Ibid., para. 2.12, p. 15.

70   Ibid., p. vi.

71   Department of Health, 1994, p. 41.

72   Ibid.

73   Slevin, 1989, pp. 27–30.

74   Simons, *et al.*, 1998, p. 14.

75   Ibid., p. 46.

76   Ibid., p. 48.

77   Anon., 1994, pp. 22–5.

78   For a discussion on the 'clinical practice ethic', see Bradshaw, 2001, pp. 215–16.

79   The programme attracted an initial 2, 000 applications, of which 1,600 satisfied the entry requirements. Selection was based on an interview. See Anon., 1994, pp. 22–5.

80   'Editorial', *An Bord Altranais News*, 1994, vol. 6 (3), p. 1.

81   Simons, *et al.*, 1998, p. 14.

82   'Editorial', *An Bord Altranais News*, 1994, vol. 6 (3), p. 1.

83   Ibid.

84   Madden, 1994, p. 7. See also Simons, *et al.*, 1998, p. 14.

85   An Bord Altranais, 1994b, p. 12.

86   Madden, 1994, p. 7.

87   Clarke, 1996.

88   The Department's directives were set out in a series of internal confidential departmental memoranda.

89   Fealy, 2004a, pp. 43–54.

90   Bradshaw, 2001, pp. 231–6.

91   Simons, *et al.*, 1998, p. 39.

92   An Bord Altranais, 1991b, p. 5.

93   Akinsanya, 1990, pp. 744–54.

94   Hyde and Treacy, 2000, pp. 89–108.

95   Ibid., p. 89.

9 Conclusions

1 I am grateful to Dr Deirdre Raftery, Education Department, University College Dublin, for her helpful suggestions in this regard.
2 Rosenberg asks if the nurse's relation to medical knowledge raised or permanently limited her status. See Rosenberg, 1987, pp. 67–8.
3 Fealy, 2004b, pp. 649–56.
4 Ibid., p. 652.
5 Ibid.
6 Government of Ireland, *Report of the Commission on Nursing: A Blueprint for the Future*, Dublin: The Stationery Office, 1998.
7 Chavasse, 1998, vol. 28, pp. 172–7.
8 Cowman, 2001, pp. 419–20.
9 Government of Ireland, 1998, p. 3.

References

Abel-Smith, B., 1960, *A History of the Nursing Profession*, London: Heinemann.

Acts of the Oireachtas, 1950, *The Nurses Act 1950*, No. 27, Dublin: The Stationery Office.

——, 1985, *The Nurses Act 1985*, Dublin: The Stationery Office.

Akinsanya, J.,1990, 'Nursing links with higher education: a prescription for change in the 21st century', *Journal of Advanced Nursing*, vol. 15, pp. 744–54.

An Bord Altranais, 1953, *Nurses Rules 1953*, Dublin: An Bord Altranais.

——, 1955, *Regulations and Guides to the Minimum Conditions which must exist before a Hospital or Training Institution is Approved by above Board*, Dublin: An Bord Altranais.

——, 1973, Memorandum on Nurses Standards of General Education, Dublin: An Bord Altranais.

——, 1979, *Syllabus of Training for Registered General Nurses*, Dublin: An Bord Altranais.

——, 1980, *Guidelines to the Implementation of the Syllabus of Training for Registered General Nurses*, Dublin: An Bord Altranais.

——, 1987, *Newsletter*, vol. 4 (1).

——, 1991a, *Rules and Criteria for the Education and Training of Student Nurses*, Dublin: An Bord Altranais.

——, 1991b, *Nurse Education and Training Consultative Document: Interim Report of the Review Committee*, Dublin: An Bord Altranais

——, 1994a, *The Future of Nurse Education and Training in Ireland*, Dublin: An Bord Altranais.

——, 1994b, *Report for the Year 1994*, Dublin: An Bord Altranais.

——, undated a, *Syllabus of Courses of Instruction*, Dublin: An Bord Altranais.

——, undated b, *Record Charts of Practical Nursing Instruction and Experience for the Certificate of General, Infectious Disease and Sick Children's Nursing*, Dublin: An Bord Altranais.

Anderson, J., 1897, *Notes on Medical Nursing: From the Lectures Given to the Probationers at the London Hospital* (edited by E. L. Lamport), London: H. K. Lewis.

Anon., 1892, 'The Hospitals of Dublin: No. 4. – The City of Dublin Hospital', *The Lady of the House*, 14 April.

——, 1894, 'The nurses of the Irish hospitals, No. II. – The City of Dublin Nursing Institute', *The Lady of the House*, 15 December.

——, 1895a, 'The nurses of the Irish hospitals, No. III. – Adelaide Hospital nursing school', *The Lady of the House*, 15 January.

——, 1895b, 'The nurses of the Irish hospitals', No. III. – St Patrick's Home for supplying trained nurses to the sick poor in their own homes', *The Lady of the House*, 15 February.

——, 1895c, 'The nurses of the Irish hospitals, No. V. – The nurses of the Mater Misericordiae Hospital', *The Lady of the House*, 15 March.

——, 1895d, 'The nurses of the Irish hospitals: No. VI. – the lady nurses of the Red Cross', *The Lady of the House*, 15 April.

——, 1985e, 'The nurses of the Irish hospitals, No. VI. – The lady nurses of Sir Patrick Dun's Hospital', *The Lady of the House*, 15 May.

——, 1895f, 'The nurses of the Irish hospitals; No. VIII. – Nursing school at Cork Street Fever Hospital', *The Lady of the House*, 15 June.

——, 1895g, 'The nurses of the Irish hospitals, No. X. – The nurses of Jervis Street Hospital', *The Lady of the House*, 14 September.

——, 1895h, 'The nurses of the Irish Hospitals, No. XI. – nursing school of Dr Steevens' Hospital', *The Lady of the House*, 15 October.

——, 1896a 'The lady nurses of the Irish hospitals; No. XIII. – Dublin Nurses' Training Institution, 26 Usher's Quay, Dublin', *The Lady of the House*, 15 January.

——, 1896b, 'The nurses of the Irish hospitals, No. XIV. – The school of St Vincent's Hospital', *The Lady of the House*, 15 February.

——, 1896c, 'The nurses of the Irish Hospitals, No. XV. – Nursing school of the Royal Hospital for Incurables, Donnybrook', *The Lady of the House*, 14 March.

——, 1896d, 'The nurses of the Irish hospitals', No. XVI. – Nursing School of the Richmond, Hardwicke and Whitworth Hospitals, North Brunswick Street, *The Lady of the House*, 15 June .

——, 1902, 'The lady superintendents of the Irish hospitals', *The Lady of the House*, Christmas.

——, 1909, 'The first lady nurse trained in Ireland to become a Hospital Superintendent', *The Lady of the House*, 15 April.

——, 1966, 'Desirable of improving conditions for student nurses', *Irish Nursing and Hospital World*, vol. 37 (6), pp. 9–10.

——, 1994, 'New pilot project in the education and training of student nurses', *An Bord Altranais News*, vol. 6 (3), pp. 22–5.

Arden, P., 2002, *When Matron Ruled*, London: Robert Hale.

Baly, M. E., 1977, *Nursing*, London: B. T. Batsford Ltd.

——, 1987, *A History of the Queen's Nursing Institute*, Beckenham: Croom Helm. Ltd.

——, 1995, *Nursing and Social Change* (Third Edition), London: Routledge.

Banks, J. T., 1883, Richmond, Whitworth, and Hardwicke Government Hospitals: Introductory Address Delivered to the Opening of the Medical Session, 1st November, Dublin: Gunn and Cameron.

Barber, J. A., 1998, 'Uniform and nursing reform', *International History of Nursing Journal*, vol. 3 (1), pp. 20–9

Barrington, R., 1987, *Health, Medicine and Politics in Ireland 1900–1970*, Dublin: Institute of Public Administration.

Basford, L., 1995, 'Precedents', in L. Basford and O. Slevin (eds), *Theory and Practice of Nursing: An Integrated Approach to Patient Care*, Edinburgh: Campion Press, pp. 25–48.

Baubérot, J., 1993, 'The Protestant woman', in G. Fraisse and M. Perrot (eds), *A History of Women in the West: IV Emerging Feminism from Revolution to World War*, Cambridge: The Belknap Press. pp. 198–212.

Bendall, E. R. D., 1975, *So You Passed Nurse*, London: Royal College of Nursing and National Council of Nurses of the United Kingdom.

Bennett, P., 1986, 'Diary feature: a week in the life of a student nurse', *Nursing Review*, vol. 4 (1 and 2), p. 20.

Boland, P., 1957, 'The preliminary training school: an appreciation', *St. Vincent's Hospital Annual: The Mary Aikenhead School of Nursing*, Dublin: St. Vincent's Hospital.

Bolster, E., 1964, *The Sisters of Mercy in the Crimean War*, Dublin: The Mercier Press.

Borer, M. C., 1975, *Willingly to School: A History of Women's Education*, Guilford: Lutterworth Press.

Bradshaw, A., 2001, *The Nurse Apprentice, 1860–1977*, Aldershot: Ashgate.

Breathnach, E., 1987, 'Charting new waters: women's experience in higher education, 1879–1908', in M. Cullen (ed.), *Girls Don't Do Honours: Irish Women in Education in the 19th and 20th Centuries*, Dublin: Women's Education Bureau.

Broe, E.,1955, 'New trends in nursing education', *The Irish Nurses' Magazine*, vol. 22 (6), pp. 10–2 and vol. 22 (7), pp. 12–4.

Brooks, J., 2001, 'Structured by class, bound by gender', *International History of Nursing Journal*, vol. 6 (2), pp. 13–21

Burke, H., 1987, *The People and the Poor Law in 19th Century Ireland*, Dublin: The Women's Education Bureau.

Cantlie, J., 1914, *British Red Cross Society Nursing Manual No 2*, London: Cassell and Company, Ltd.

Chavasse, J., 1968, 'Nursing in the Emerald Isle', *International Nursing Review*, vol. 15 (3), pp. 182–8.

——, 1998, 'Policy as an influence on public health nursing education in the Republic of Ireland', *Journal of Advanced Nursing*, vol. 28, pp. 172–7.

——, 2000, 'Nursing education', in J. Robins (ed.), *Nursing and Midwifery in Ireland in the Twentieth Century*, Dublin: An Bord Altranais, pp. 197–212.

City of Dublin Hospital, 1879, *Forty-seventh Report of the City of Dublin Hospital, Upper Baggot Street for the Year 1878*, Dublin: City of Dublin Hospital.

——, 1880, *Forty-eighth Report of the City of Dublin Hospital, Upper Baggot Street for the Year 1879*, Dublin: City of Dublin Hospital.

——, 1884a, *Fifty-second Report of the City of Dublin Hospital, Upper Baggot Street for the Year 1883*, Dublin: City of Dublin Hospital.

——, 1884b, *City of Dublin Nursing Institution Limited, (in Connection with the City of Dublin Hospital) Regulations of the Institution and Probationers' Application for Admission Engagement of Nurse and Rules*, (Insert in Board of Directors Minute Book, 8 February 1884).

——, 1884c, *Board of Directors Minute Book, City of Dublin Hospital*, Dublin: City of Dublin Hospital.

——, 1884d *City of Dublin Hospital and City of Dublin Nursing Institution Limited, Upper Baggot Street Dublin: The Lady Superintendent* (Insert in Board of Directors Minute Book, 22 February 1884).

——, 1885, *Fifty-third Report of the City of Dublin Hospital, Upper Baggot Street for the Year 1884*, Dublin: City of Dublin Hospital.

——, 1886, *Fifty-fourth Report of the City of Dublin Hospital, Upper Baggot Street for the Year 1885*, Dublin: City of Dublin Hospital.

——, 1887, *Fifty-fifth Report of the City of Dublin Hospital, Upper Baggot Street for the Year 1886*, Dublin: City of Dublin Hospital.

——, 1888, *Fifty-sixth Report of the City of Dublin Hospital, Upper Baggot Street for the Year 1887*, Dublin: City of Dublin Hospital.

——, 1892, *Sixtieth Report of The City of Dublin Hospital, Upper Baggot Street for the Year 1891*, Dublin: City of Dublin Hospital.

——, 1894, *Sixty-third Report of the City of Dublin Hospital, Upper Baggot Street for the Year 1893*, Dublin: City of Dublin Hospital.

——, 1903, *Seventy-first Report of the City of Dublin Hospital, Upper Baggot Street for the Year 1902*, Dublin: City of Dublin Hospital.

——, 1911, *Seventy-ninth Report of the City of Dublin Hospital, Upper Baggot Street for the Year 1910*, Dublin: City of Dublin Hospital.

Clarke, D. J., 1996, 'Where to from here? – The emerging issues', *Proceedings, Association of Nurse Teachers Conference*, Dublin: Association of Nurse Teachers.

Clear, C., 1987, *Nuns in Nineteenth-century Ireland*, Dublin: Gill and McMillan.

Clery, A. B., 1972, 'Nursing in the House of Industry Hospitals', in Widdess, *The Richmond, Whitworth and Hardwicke Hospitals. St Laurence's Hospital, Dublin, 1772–1972*, Dublin: Beacon Printing, pp. 155–63.

Coakley, D., 1995, *Baggot Street: A Short History of the Royal City of Dublin Hospital*, Dublin: Royal City of Dublin Hospital Board of Governors.

Coey Bigger, E., 1937, 'The training and registration of nurses', *The Irish Free State Hospital Yearbook and Medical Directory* (First Edition), Dublin: O'Neill Publications Ltd.

Connolly, B. and Ryan, A. B. (eds), 2000, *Women and Education in Ireland: Volume 1*, Maynooth: Mace.

Costello, M., 1897, 'A tribute to Dublin nursing', *Lady of the House*, 15 November.

Counihan, H., 1951, 'The health of student nurses', *The Irish Journal of Medical Science*, Sixth Series, No. 307, pp. 304–15.

Cowman, S., 1989, 'Nurse education in Ireland 1989: present and future perspectives', *Nursing Review*, vol. 7 (3 & 4), pp. 25–7.

——, 1990 'Response to paper on nurse education proposals for reform', *Invitational Conference on Nurse Education*, Dublin, 7–8 June 1990, pp. 53–8.

——, 2001, 'Nursing education in Ireland: the end of the beginning and the envy of others in Europe', *Journal of Advanced Nursing*, vol. 34, pp. 419–20.

Culhane, M. M., 1952, 'Speaking of things', *Irish Nursing News*, August–September.

—— and Luddy, M., 1995, *Women, Power and Consciousness in 19th Century Ireland*, Dublin: Attic Press.

D'Antonio, P., 1997, 'Nineteenth century nursing', Reflections, vol. 23 (3), pp. 16–7.

Daly, M. E., 1981, *Social and Economic History of Ireland Since 1800*, Dublin: The Educational Company.

——, 1984, *Dublin: The Deposed Capital: A Social and Economic History 1860–1914*, Cork: Cork University Press.

——, 1999, 'An atmosphere of sturdy independence': the State and the Dublin hospitals in the 1930s', in E. Malcolm and G. Jones (eds), *Medicine Disease and the State in Ireland 1650–1940*, Cork: Cork University Press.

Davies, C., 1995, *Gender and Professional Predicament in Nursing*, Buckingham: Open University Press.

Davies, E., 1987, 'Home and the higher education (1878)', in D. Spender (ed.), *The Education Papers: Women's Quest for Equality in Britain 1850–1912*, London: Routledge and Kegan Paul, pp. 111–22.

Dean, M. and Bolton, G., 1980, 'The administration of poverty and the development of nursing practice in nineteenth-century England', in C. Davies (ed.), *Rewriting Nursing History*, London: Croom Helm, pp. 76–101.

Deeny, J., 1949, 'Lecture', *The Irish Nurses' Magazine*, vol. 16 (11), pp. 2–5.

——, 1989, *To Cure and to Care: Memoirs of a Chief Medical Officer*, Dublin: The Glendale Press.

Denny, E., 1997, 'The second missing link: Bible nursing in 19th century London', *Journal of Advanced Nursing*, vol. 26, pp. 1175–82.

Department of Health, 1980, *Working Party on General Nursing*, Dublin: The Stationery Office.

——, 1986, *Health – the Wider Dimensions*, Dublin: The Stationery Office.

——, 1994, *Shaping a Healthier Future: a Strategy for Effective Healthcare in the 1990s*, Dublin: The Stationery Office.

Digby, A. and Searby, A., 1981, *Children, School and Society in Nineteenth Century England*, London: The Macmillan Press Ltd.

Dingwall, R., Rafferty, A. M. and Webster, C., 1988, *An Introduction to the Social History of Nursing*, London: Routledge.

Doona, M. E., 1995, 'Sister Mary Joseph Croke: another voice from the Crimean War, 1854–1856', *Nursing History Review*, vol. 3, pp. 3–41.

——, June 1999, 'The Confidential Report on Crimean Nursing', *International Council of Nursing Centennial Conference, Celebrating Nursing's Past: Reclaiming the Future*, London.

Drew, M., 1889, *Hints on Nursing*, London: R. Forder.

Dublin Hospital Sunday Fund, 1875, *Annual Report of the Council for the Year 1874, with List of Council and Officers, Rules for the Management of the Fund for the Year 1875 and List of Collections and Subscriptions for 1874*, Dublin: Browne and Nolan.

——, 1876, *Annual Report of the Council for the Year 1875, with List of Council and Officers, Rules for the Management of the Fund for the Year 1876 and List of Collections and Subscriptions for 1875*, Dublin: Browne and Nolan.

——, 1879, *Annual Report of the Council for the Year 1878, with List of Council and Officers, Rules for the Management of the Fund for the Year 1879 and List of Collections and Subscriptions for 1878, (containing Report on the Nursing Arrangements in the Hospitals Receiving Aid from the Dublin Hospitals Sunday Fund)*, Dublin: Browne and Nolan.

——, 1880, *Annual Report of the Council for the Year 1879, with List of Council and Officers, Rules for the Management of the Fund for the Year 1880 and List of Collections and Subscriptions for 1879*, Dublin: Browne and Nolan.

——, 1881, *Annual Report of the Council for the Year 1880, with List of Council and Officers, Rules for the Management of the Fund for the Year 1881 and List of Collections and Subscriptions for 1880*, Dublin: Browne and Nolan.

——, 1883, *Report of the Council and Statement of Accounts, with List of Collections and Subscriptions for the Year 1882*, Dublin: Browne and Nolan.

——, 1887, *Report of the Council and Statement of Accounts, with List of Collections and Subscriptions for the Year 1886*, Dublin: Browne and Nolan.

——, 1888, *Report of the Council and Statement of Accounts, with List of Collections and Subscriptions for the Year 1887*, Dublin: Browne and Nolan.

——, 1889, *Report of the Council and Statement of Accounts, with List of Collections and Subscriptions for the Year 1888*, Dublin: Browne and Nolan.

——, 1931, *Report for the Year 1930–1931, (Collections for the Year 1929–1930)*, Dublin: Browne and Nolan.

Dublin House of Industry Hospitals, 1894, *Minutes of Proceedings of the Board of Governors, Dublin House of Industry Hospitals*, Dublin: DHIH, 10 August 1871–4 October 1894.

Dwyer, M. and P. Taaffe, 1997, 'Nursing in 21st century Ireland: opportunities for transformation', in A. L. Leahy and M. A. Wiley (eds), *The Irish Health System in the 21st Century*, Dublin: Oak Tree Press, pp. 237–52.

Elms, R. R., B. Tierney and P. A. Boylan, 1974, 'Irish nursing at the crossroads', *International Journal of Nursing Studies*, vol. 11, pp. 163–72.

Fahey, T., 1987, 'Nuns in the Catholic Church in Ireland in the nineteenth century', in M. Cullen (ed.), *Girls Don't Do Honours: Irish Women in Education in the 19th and 20th Centuries*, Dublin: Women's Education Bureau.

——, 1988, 'The Catholic Church and social policy', in S. Healy and B. Reynolds (eds), *Social Policy in Ireland: Principles, Practice and Problems*, Dublin: Oak Tree Press, pp. 411–29.

Fealy, G. M., 1997, 'The theory-practice relationship in nursing: an exploration of contemporary discourse', *Journal of Advanced Nursing*, vol. 25, pp. 1061–69.

——, 2004a, 'A New Era Begins, 1994–2004', in M. Duff, G. Fealy, I. Smyth, (eds), *Nursing Education in Drogheda, 1946–2004*: A Commemorative History, Drogheda: The Nursing Education Commemorative Committee.

——, 2004b, 'The good nurse': visions and values in images of the nurse', *Journal of Advanced Nursing*, vol. 64, (5), pp. 649–56.

——, 2005, 'A place for the better technical education of nurses': the Dublin Metropolitan Technical School for Nurses, 1893–1969' *Nursing History Review*, vol. 13, pp. 23–47.

Fleetwood, J., 1951, *History of Medicine in Ireland*, Dublin: Browne and Nolan Ltd.

Francis, K., 2001, 'Service to the poor: the foundations of community nursing in England, Ireland and New South Wales', *International Journal of Nursing Practice*, vol. 7, pp. 169–76.

Gamarnikow, E., 1991, 'Nurse or woman: gender and professionalism in reformed nursing, 1860–1923', in P. Holden and J. Littlewood (eds), *Anthropology and Nursing*, London: Routledge.

Gatenby, P., 1996, *Dublin's Meath Hospital 1753–1996*, Dublin: Town House.

General Nursing Council for Ireland, 1920, *Rules Made Under Nurses' Registration (Ireland) Act 1919*, Dublin: General Nursing Council for Ireland.

General Nursing Council for Ireland, 1920–1943, *Minutes of General Nursing Council for Ireland*, Dublin: GNCI.

——, 1923, *Regulations Made by the General Nursing Council for the Recognition of Hospitals as Training Schools for Nurses, Dublin: John Falconer.*

——, 1931, *Regulations made by the General Nursing Council for the Recognition of Hospitals as Training Schools for Nurses*, Dublin: George Hughes & Co.

——, 1934, *Scheme for Conducting Examinations*, Dublin: George Hughes & Co.

Government of Ireland, 1949, *The Nurses Bill*, Dublin: The Stationery Office.

——, 1998, *Report of the Commission on Nursing: A Blueprint for the Future*, Dublin: The Stationery Office.

Griffon, D. P., 1995, '"Crowning the edifice": Ethel Fenwick and State Registration', *Nursing History Review*, vol. 3, pp. 201–12.

Hanrahan, E., 1970, *Report on the Training of Student Nurses*, Dublin: Irish Matrons' Association.

Hector, W., 1973, *The Work of Mrs Bedford Fenwick and the Rise of Professional Nursing*, London: Royal College of Nursing.

Helmstadter, C., 1993a, 'Robert Bentley Todd, St John's House, and the origins of the modern trained nurse', *Bulletin of the History of Medicine*, vol. 67, pp. 282–319.

——, 1993b, 'Old nurses for new: nursing in the London teaching hospitals before and after the mid-nineteenth century reforms', *Nursing History Review*, vol. 1, pp. 43–70.

——, 1997, 'Doctors and nurses in the London teaching hospitals: class, gender, religion and professional expertise, 1850–1890', *Nursing History Review*, vol. 5, p. 161–97.

——, 2001, 'From the private to the public sphere: the first generation of lady nurses in England', *Nursing History Review*, vol. 9, pp. 127–40.

——, 2003, '"A real tone": professionalizing nursing in nineteenth-century London', *Nursing History Review*, vol. 11, pp. 2–30.

House of Commons, 1838, *Bill for the More Effectual Relief of the Destitute Poor in Ireland*. H.C., London: HMSO.

——, 1854, *Report of the Select Committee on Dublin Hospitals, Minutes of Evidence, Appendix and Index*, Dublin: HMSO.

——, 1856, *Report of the Commissioners Appointed to Inquire into the Hospitals of Dublin, with Appendices*, Dublin: HMSO.

——, 1858, *First Annual Report of the Board of Superintendence of Dublin Hospitals, with Appendices*, Dublin: HMSO.

——, 1862, *Act for the Relief of Destitute Poor in Ireland*, London: HMSO.

——, 1887a, *Dublin Hospitals Commission: Report of the Committee of Inquiry together with Minutes of Evidence and Appendices*, Dublin: HMSO.

——, 1887b, *Bill to Provide for a Dublin Hospital Board*, Dublin: HMSO.

——, 1889, *Bill for the Establishment of a Dublin Hospital Board*, Dublin: HMSO.

——, 1890, *Thirty-second Report of the Board of Superintendence of Dublin Hospitals, with Appendices*, Dublin: HMSO.

——, 1892, *Thirty-fourth Report of the Board of Superintendence of Dublin Hospitals, with Appendices*, Dublin: HMSO.

——, 1899, *Forty-first Report of the Board of Superintendence of Dublin Hospitals, with Appendices*, Dublin: HMSO.

——, 1904a, *Select Committee on the Registration of Nurses, together with the Proceedings of the Committee, Minutes of Evidence, Appendix and Index*, London: HMSO.

——, 1904b, *Bill to Regulate the Qualification of Trained Nurses and to Provide for their Registration*, London: HMSO.

——, 1919a, *Bill to Provide for the State Registration of Nurses in Ireland*, Dublin: HMSO.

——, 1919b, *Nurses Registration (Ireland) Act*, Dublin: HMSO.

House, H., 1987, 'Introduction', in C. Dickens, *The Adventures of Oliver Twist*, Oxford: Oxford University Press.

Hyde, A. and M. Treacy, 2000, 'Nurse education in the Republic of Ireland: negotiating a new educational space', in B. Connolly, and A. B. Ryan (eds), *Women and Education in Ireland: Volume 1*, Maynooth: Mace, pp. 89–108.

Jex-Blake, S., 1987, 'The medical education of women (1873)', in D. Spender (ed.), *The Education Papers*, pp. 268–76.

Kelly, J., 1999, 'The emergence of scientific institutional medical practice in Ireland, 1650–1880', in Malcolm and Jones, *Medicine, Disease and the State in Ireand, 1850–1940*, Cork: Cork University Press, pp. 21–39.

Kelly, P., 1972, From Workhouse to Hospital: the Role of the Irish Workhouse in medical relief to 1921, Unpublished M.A. Thesis, Galway: University College Galway.

Kirkpatrick, T. C P., 1917a, *Nursing Ethics: A Lecture*, Dublin: The University Press.

——, 1917b, *Registration for Nurses: A Lecture Delivered in the Dublin Metropolitan Technical School for Nurses*, Dublin: University Press.

——, 1924, *History of Dr Steevens' Hospital Dublin: 1720–1920*, Dublin: University Press.

Knibiehler, Y., 1993, 'Bodies and Hearts', in G. Fraisse and M. Perrot (eds), *A History of Women in the West: IV Emerging Feminism from Revolution to World War*, Cambridge: The Belknap Press, pp. 325–68.

Lennon, Sr M. I., 1960, 'Nursing: Ireland v. United States', *The Irish Nurses' Magazine*, vol. 27 (11), pp. 3–7.

Lewenson, S., 1994, '"Of logical necessity … they hang together": nursing and the women's movement 1901–1912', *Nursing History Review*, vol. 2, pp. 99–117.

Leydon, I., 1972, 'Future trends in nursing', *World of Irish Nursing*, vol. 1 (5), pp. 101–2.

——, 1979, 'Implications for the EEC Directives on general nurse training', *World of Irish Nursing*, vol. 8 (1 and 2).

Lorentzon, M., 2001, 'Grooming nurses for the new century: analysis of nurses' registers in London voluntary hospitals before the First World War', *International History of Nursing Journal*, vol. 6 (2), pp. 4–12.

——, 2003, 'Socialising nurse probationers in the late 19th and early 20th centuries – relevance of historical reflection for modern policy makers', *Nurse Education Today*, vol. 23, pp. 325–31.

Lückes, E. C. E., 1892, *Lectures on General Nursing*, London: Kegan Paul, Trench, Trübner & Co.

——, 1886, *Hospital Sisters and their Duties* (First Edition), London: J. & A. Churchill.

Luddy, M., 1995, *Women and Philanthropy in Nineteenth-century Ireland*, Cambridge: Cambridge University Press.

——, 1997, *Women in Ireland 1800–1918: A Documentary History*, Cork: Cork University Press.

——, 1999, '"Angels of Mercy": Nuns as Workhouse Nurses', in E. Malcolm and G. Jones (eds), *Medicine, Disease and the State in Ireland 1650–1940*, Cork: Cork University Press, pp. 102–17.

MacGuire, J., 1968, 'The functions of the set in hospital controlled schemes of nurse training', *British Journal of Sociology*, vol. 19, pp. 271–82.

MacLurg Jensen, D., 1959, *History and Trends of Professional Nursing* (Fourth Edition), St Louis: C. V. Mosby Co.

McCarthy, G., 1989, *Student Nurses in the Republic of Ireland: A Study of their Biographical, Educational, Motivational and Personality Characteristics*, Unpublished Master of Education Thesis, Dublin: University of Dublin, Trinity College Dublin.

——, 1990a, 'Nurse education: proposals for reform', *World of Irish Nursing*, November/December, pp. 5–14.

——, 1990b, 'Nurse education: proposals for reform', *Invitational Conference on Nurse Education* (hosted by Case Western Reserve University, Ohio USA and University College Galway), Dublin, 7 and 8 June .

McGann, S., 1992, *The Battle of the Nurses: A Study of Eight Women who Influenced the Development of Professional Nursing, 1880–1930*, London: Scutari Press.

McGeachie, J., 1999, '"Normal" development in an "Abnormal" place, Sir William Wilde and the Irish School of Medicine', in E. Malcolm and G. Jones (eds), *Medicine Disease and the State in Ireland 1850-1940*, Cork: Cork University Press, pp. 85–101.

McGowan, J., 1980, *Attitude Survey of Irish Nurses*, Dublin: Institute of Public Administration.

McNamara, Sr C., 1987, 'The continuous nurse learner', *Nursing Review*, vol. 6 (1), pp. 3–5.

McNeill, M., 1934, 'The nursing school', in Anon., *A Century of Service*, Dublin: Browne and Nolan.

McShane, S., 1999, *Hidden aspects of nursing inequality: a documentary analysis of health policy development and implementation during the period 1945–1994*, Unpublished Master of Equality Studies Thesis, Dublin: University College Dublin.

Madden, P. J., 1994, 'The future education and training of nurses', *The New World of Irish Nursing*, vol. 2 (4).

Maillart, V., 1973, 'Higher education in nursing', *Irish Nursing News*, vol. 154, pp. 13–6.

Mater Misericordiae Hospital, 1961, 'College of Nursing', *Mater Misericordiae Hospital Centenary 1861–1961: Commemorative Brochure*, Dublin: Parkside Press Ltd.

Meehan, T. C., 2003, 'Careful nursing: a model for contemporary nursing practice', *Journal of Advanced Nursing*, vol. 44 (1), pp. 99–107.

Melia, K. M., 1987, *Learning and Working: The Occupational Socialisation of Nurses*, London: Tavistock.

Menzies Lyth, I., 2000, 'Social systems as a defence against anxiety', in E. Trist and H. Murray (eds), *The Social Engagement of Social Science, Volume 1: The Socio-Psychological Perspective*, London: Free Association Books, pp. 439–62.

Millard, M.,1944, 'Trinity College meeting', *Irish Nurses' Magazine*, vol. 13 (37), pp. 6–8.

Mitchell, D., 1989, *A 'Peculiar' Place: the Adelaide Hospital, Dublin, its Times, Places and Personalities 1839–1989*, Dublin: Blackwater.

Murray, Reverend Father P. 1968, 'The Sisters of Mercy at Jervis Street Hospital', in J. D. H. Widdess, *The Charitable Infirmary, Jervis Street, Dublin, 1718–1968*, Dublin: The Charitable Infirmary Jervis Street.

Nelson, S., 1997, 'Pastoral care and moral government: early nineteenth century nursing and solutions to the Irish question', *Journal of Advanced Nursing*, vol. 26, pp. 6–14.

——, 1999, 'Entering the professional domain: the making of the modern nurse in 17th century France', *Nursing History Review*, vol. 7. pp. 171–87.

——, 2001, *Say Little, Do Much: Nursing, Nuns, and Hospitals in the Nineteenth Century*, Philadelphia: University of Pennsylvania Press,.

Nightingale, F., 1969, *Notes on Nursing: What it is and What it is Not* (Facsimile of the 1860 Edition), New York: Dover Publications Inc.

Nolan, M. E., 1991, *One Hundred Years: A History of the School of Nursing and of Developments at the Mater Misericordiae Hospital 1891–1991*, Dublin: Congregation of the Sisters of Mercy.

O'Brien, E., 1984, 'The Georgian Era, 1714–1835', in E. O'Brien, A. Crookshank and G. Wolstenholme (eds), *A Portrait of Irish Medicine: An Illustrated History of Medicine in Ireland*, Dublin: Ward River Press, pp. 75–114.

——, 1988, 'Of vagabonds, sturdy beggars and strolling women', in E. O'Brien, L. Browne and K. O' Malley (eds), *The House of Industry Hospitals: 1772–1987: The Richmond, Whitworth and Hardwicke (St Laurence's Hospital): A Closing Memoir*, Dublin: The Anniversary Press.

O'Brien, E., Crookshank, A. and Wolstenholme, G. (eds), 1984, *A Portrait of Irish Medicine: An Illustrated History of Medicine in Ireland*, Dublin: Ward River Press.

O'Connor, A. V., 1987. 'The revolution in girl's secondary education in Ireland, 1860–1910', in M. Cullen (ed.), *Girls Don't Do Honours: Irish Women in Education in the 19th and 20th Centuries*, Dublin: Women's Education Bureau.

——, 1995, 'Anne Jellicoe', in M. Cullen and M. Luddy, *Women, Power and Consciousness in 19th Century Ireland*, Dublin: Attic Press.

Oakley, A., 1993, *Essays on Women, Medicine and Health*, Edinburgh: Edinburgh University Press.

Pearson, A., H. Baker, K. Walsh and M. Fitzgerald, 2001, 'Contemporary nurses' uniforms – history and traditions', *Journal of Nursing Management*, vol. 9, pp. 147–52.

Pincoffs, M. C., 1893, *What Constitutes an Efficient Nurse and Other Papers*, London: The Record Press Ltd.

Preston, M., 1998, 'The good nurse: women philanthropists and the evolution of nursing in Dublin', *New Hibernia Review*, vol. 2 (1), pp. 91–110.

Purvis, J., 1989, *Hard Lessons: The Lives and Education of Working-class Women in Nineteenth-Century England*, Cambridge: Polity Press.

Quinn, S., 1980, 'The EEC directives on training in nursing', in S. Quinn (ed.), *Nursing in the European Community*, London: Croom Helm, pp. 168–76.

Rafferty, A. M., 1991, *The Politics of Nurse Education 1860–1948*, Ph.D. Thesis, Oxford: Oxford University (Bodleian).

——, 1993, 'Decorous didactics: early explorations in the art and science of caring', in A. Kitson (ed.), *Nursing Art and Science*, London: Chapman Hall, pp. 48–60.

——, 1995, 'The anomaly of autonomy: space and status in early nursing reform', *International History of Nursing Journal*, vol. 1 (1), pp. 43–56.

——, 1996, *The Politics of Nursing Knowledge*, London: Routledge.

Raftery, D., 1997, *Women and Learning in English Writing, 1600–1900*, Dublin: Four Courts Press.

Reeves, A.,1940, 'An appreciation of the late Miss Margaret Huxley, R.G.N., M.A.', *British Journal of Nursing*, vol. 88, pp. 27–8.

Richmond, Whitworth and Hardwicke Hospitals, 1890, *Regulations Regarding Nursing Department*, Dublin: Richmond, Whitworth and Hardwicke Hospitals.

Richmond, Whitworth and Hardwicke Hospitals, undated, *c.*1930, *Practical Lectures According to the Syllabus of General Nursing Council for Preliminary Examination*, Dublin: Richmond, Whitworth and Hardwicke Hospitals.

Robins, J., 2000a, 'The Irish nurse in the early 1900s', in J.Robins (ed.), *Nursing and Midwifery in Ireland in the Twentieth Century*, Dublin: An Bord Altranais.

——, 2000b, 'An Bord Altranais. 1950–1970', in J. Robins (ed.), *Nursing and Midwifery in Ireland in the Twentieth Century*, Dublin: An Bord Altranais.

——, 2000c, 'An Bord Altranais after 1970', in J. Robins (ed.), *Nursing and Midwifery in Ireland in the Twentieth Century*, Dublin: An Bord Altranais, p. 57.

Romanes, G. J., 1987, 'Mental differences between men and women, (1887)', in D. Spender (ed.), *The Education Papers*.

Rose, Sr Frances, 1957, 'Nurse education today', *St. Vincent's Hospital Dublin Annual*, Dublin: St. Vincent's Hospital.

Rosenberg, C. C., 1987, 'Clio and caring: an agenda for American historians and nursing', *Nursing Research*, vol. 36 (1) pp. 67–8.

Royal City of Dublin Hospital, 1920, *Nursing Committee Minute Book*, Dublin: RCDH

Royal City of Dublin Hospital, 1975, Report 1969–1975, Dublin: Royal City of Dublin Hospital.

Rumsey, H. W., 1873, *The Training of Nurses: a Paper* (read at the Annual General Assembly of the Order of St John of Jerusalem, held in London on St John Baptist's Day).

Russell, S., 1980, 'The European ideal', in S. Quinn, (ed.), *Nursing in the European Community*, London: Croom Helm.

Ryan, A. M., 2000, 'General nursing', in Robins, *Nursing and Midwifery in Ireland in the Twentieth Century*, Dublin: An Bord Altranais.

S. M. C., 1961, 'The right approach to hospital discipline', in Mater Misericordiae Hospital, *College of Nursing Commemorative Brochure*.

Scanlan, P., 1966, '*Nursing Education in Ireland: Background, Present Status, and Future*', unpublished PhD thesis, Washington: The Catholic University of America , pp. 356–7.

——, 1969, 'Nursing education in Ireland', *International Nursing Review*, vol. 16 (2), pp. 153–60.

——, 1991, *The Irish Nurse: A Study of Nursing in Ireland: History and Education, 1718–1981*, Manorhamilton: Drumlin.

Scott, J. W., 1993, 'The woman worker', in G. Fraisse and M. Perrot (eds), *A History of Women in the West: IV Emerging Feminism from Revolution to World War*, Cambridge: The Belknap Press, pp. 399–426.

Sears, W. G., 1941, *Anatomy and Physiology for Nurses and Students of Human Biology*, London: Edward Arnold Publishers Ltd.

Simonton, D., 2001, 'Nursing history as women's history', *International History of Nursing Journal*, vol. 6 (1), pp. 35–47.

Simons, H., J. B. Clarke, M. Gobbi and G. Long, 1998, *Nurse Education and Training Evaluation in Ireland*, Dublin: Department of Health.

Simpson, H. M., 1968, 'Satisfaction and dissatisfaction of student life', *International Nursing Review*, vol. 15 (4), pp. 329–38.

Sir Patrick Dun's Hospital, 1945, *Report of Sir Patrick Dun's Hospital, Year Ended 31st December 1944*, Dublin: Sir Patrick Dun's Hospital.

——, 1946, *Report of Sir Patrick Dun's Hospital, Year Ended 31st December 1945*, Dublin: Sir Patrick Dun's Hospital.

Slater, V. E., 1994, 'The educational and philosophical influences of Florence Nightingale, an enlightened conductor', *Nursing History Review* vol. 2, pp. 137–52.

Slevin, O., 1989, 'Project 2000: towards implementation in Northern Ireland', *Nursing Standard*, vol. 40 (3), pp. 27–30.

Spender, D. (ed.), 1987, *The Education Papers: Women's Quest for Equality in Britain, 1850–1912*, London: Routledge and Kegan Paul.

Summers, A., 1989a, 'Ministering angels', *History Today*, vol. 39. pp. 31–7.

——, 1989b, 'The mysterious demise of Sarah Gamp: the domiciliary nurse and her detractors, c.1830–1860', *Victorian Studies*, Spring, pp. 365–86.

——, 2000, *Female Lives, Moral States: Women, Religion and Public Life in Britain, 1800–1930*, Newbury: Threshold Press.

Tierney, B., 1974 'Nursing in Ireland', *International Journal of Nursing Studies*, vol. 11, pp. 111–7.

Tod, I. S. M., 1987, 'On the education of girls of the middle classes (1874)', in Spender (ed.), *The Education Papers*, pp. 230–47.

Treacy, M. P., 1987, 'Some aspects of the hidden curriculum', in P. Allen and M. Jolly (eds), *The Curriculum in Nursing Education*, London: Croom Helm, pp. 164–75.

——, 1989, 'Gender prescription in nurse training: its effects on health care provision', *Recent Advances in Nursing*, vol. 25, pp. 70–91.

Vickery, A., 1998, 'Golden Age to Separate Spheres? A Review of the Categories and Chronology of Women's History' in P. Sharpe, (ed.), *Women's Work, the English Experience, 1650–1914*, London: Arnold.

Weir, R. I., 2000, 'Medical and nursing education in the nineteenth century: comparisons and comments', *International History of Nursing Journal*, vol. 5 (2), pp. 42–7.

White, R., 1978, *Social Change and the Development of the Nursing Profession: A Study of the Poor Law Nursing Service 1848–1948*, London: Henry Kimpton Publishers.

Whyte, J., 1971, *Church and State in Modern Ireland*, Dublin: Gill and McMillan.

Wickham, A., 2000, 'A better scheme for nursing: the influence of the Dublin Hospital Sunday Fund on nursing and nurse training in Ireland in the nineteenth century', *Conference Proceedings, Royal College of Nursing History of Nursing Society Conference*, Edinburgh, July 6–7.

——, 2001, 'A better scheme for nursing: the influence of the Dublin Hospital Sunday Fund on nursing and nurse training in Ireland in the nineteenth century', *International History of Nursing Journal*, vol. 6 (2), pp. 26–34.

——, 2005, '"She must be content to be their servant as well as their teacher": the early years of district nursing in Ireland', in G. M. Fealy, *Care to Remember: Nursing and Midwifery in Ireland*, Cork: Mercier Press, pp. 102–121.

Widdess, J. D. H., 1972, *The Richmond, Whitworth and Hardwicke Hospitals. St Laurence's Hospital, Dublin, 1772–1972*, Dublin: Beacon Printing.

Witz, A., 1992, *Professions and Patriarchy*, London: Routledge.

Wolstenholme, G., 1984, 'A portrait of Irish medicine', in O'Brien, Crookshank and A Wolstenholme (eds), *A Portrait of Irish Medicine: An Illustrated History of Medicine in Ireland*, Dublin: Ward River Press, pp. 115–46.

World Health Organisation, 1985, *Targets for Health for All by the Year 2000*, Copenhagen: WHO.

Index

Printed and bound by CPI Group (UK) Ltd, Croydon, CR0 4YY

01/11/2024

01782626-0011